DIGITAL MAMMOGRAPHY

DIGITAL MAMMOGRAPHY

ETTA D. PISANO, MD, FACR

Professor of Radiology and Biomedical Engineering
Department of Radiology
University of North Carolina School of Medicine
UNC-Lineberger Comprehensive Cancer Center
Chapel Hill, North Carolina

MARTIN J. YAFFE, PhD

Senior Scientist
Imaging and Bioengineering Research
Sunnybrook & Women's College Health Sciences Centre
Professor of Medical Imaging and Medical Biophysics
University of Toronto
Toronto, Ontario, Canada

CHERIE M. KUZMIAK, DO

Assistant Professor of Radiology
Department of Radiology
University of North Carolina School of Medicine
UNC-Lineberger Comprehensive Cancer Center
Chapel Hill, North Carolina

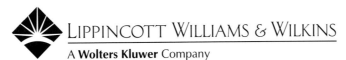

LIPPINCOTT WILLIAMS & WILKINS
A **Wolters Kluwer** Company
Philadelphia · Baltimore · New York · London
Buenos Aires · Hong Kong · Sydney · Tokyo

Acquisitions Editor: Lisa McAllister
Developmental Editor: Scott Scheidt
Supervising Editor: Mary Ann McLaughlin
Production Editor: Kathy Cleghorn, Chernow Editorial Services, Inc.
Manufacturing Manager: Ben Rivera
Cover Designer: Armen Kojoyian
Compositor: Lippincott Williams & Wilkins Desktop Division
Printer: Maple Press

© 2004 by LIPPINCOTT WILLIAMS & WILKINS
530 Walnut Street
Philadelphia, PA 19106 USA
LWW.com

Printed in the USA

Library of Congress Cataloging-in-Publication Data

Digital mammography / editors, Etta D. Pisano, Martin J. Yaffe, Cherie M. Kuzmiak.
    p. cm.
    Includes bibliographical references and index.
    ISBN 0-7817-4142-4
    1. Breast—Radiography. 2. Breast—Imaging. 3. Breast—Cancer—Diagnosis.
  I. Pisano, Etta D. II. Yaffe, Martin J. (Martin Joel), 1949– III. Kuzmiak, Cherie M.

RG493.5.R33D537 2003
618.1'907572—dc21

                                                                    2003051682

10 9 8 7 6 5 4 3 2 1

To our families, our professional mentors, and our colleagues

TABLE OF CONTENTS

CONTRIBUTING AUTHORS

Fred M. Behlen, PhD, President, LAI Technology, Homewood, Illinois

Cherie M. Kuzmiak, DO, Assistant Professor of Radiology, Department of Radiology, University of North Carolina School of Medicine, UNC-Lineberger Comprehensive Cancer Center, Chapel Hill, North Carolina

James G. Mainprize, PhD, Research Associate, Imaging Research Program, Sunnybrook & Women's College Health Sciences Centre, Toronto, Ontario, Canada

Robert M. Nishikawa, PhD, Professor of Radiology, Department of Radiology, University of Chicago, Chicago, Illinois

Etta D. Pisano, MD, FACR, Professor of Radiology and Biomedical Engineering, Department of Radiology, University of North Carolina School of Medicine, UNC-Lineberger Comprehensive Cancer Center, Chapel Hill, North Carolina

Martin J. Yaffe, PhD, Senior Scientist, Imaging and Bioengineering Research, Sunnybrook & Women's College Health Sciences Centre, and Professor of Medical Imaging and Medical Biophysics, University of Toronto, Toronto, Ontario, Canada

FOREWORD

Breast cancer is the most common and most feared cancer among women in the United States. The incidence continues to rise, and it is not entirely clear why. It is a disease of aging, as more than 75% of cases occur in women more than 50 years of age. It is second only to lung cancer as the cause of death because of a malignant disease. It receives disproportionate attention (there are 20–30 times more deaths as a result of cardiovascular disease) from not only women's groups, but also from the public at large, the media, the breast care industry, lawyers, and politicians. Costs for its detection, treatment, and follow-up are staggering.

The history of Medical Imaging (remember when it used to be called the X-ray Department!) is one of those gradual processes punctuated by a few seminal developments, such as image amplification (which eliminated the need for those "red goggles" for dark adaptation); radioisotope imaging (nuclear medicine); ultrasound imaging (sonography); computerized (digital) axial tomography (CT, or CAT, scanning); and magnetic resonance imaging (MRI). All of these techniques have been applied to breast imaging with varying degrees of success, but mammography remains the cornerstone of breast imaging. It is considered a, if not the, major means of earlier detection, thereby providing treatment options that include breast conservation and mortality reduction.

Digital imaging, especially CT, has been with us for many years and has acquired an indispensable role in examining most of the human body. The breast remains the conspicuous exception. Breast imaging is extremely demanding, especially in terms of contrast for subtle differences in soft tissue densities, and resolution for very small calcifications, margins of masses, and architectural distortions. The efficacy of screen-film mammography has delayed, if not limited, the application of digital imaging and other techniques. But its limitations also were the impetus for their continued development and clinical application.

Certainly that includes "Digital Mammography," which seems to be coming of age and is the subject of this book. The clear advantages include (1) the capacity to manipulate images; (2) Computer-assisted detection and diagnosis (CAD), including easier double or more interpretations; (3) the capacity to transmit images for consultation and other purposes, including teaching and conferences;

and (4) archiving (PACS) for simplified storage and ready access of images. Preconceived disadvantages included obstacles to change ("teaching old dogs new tricks!"), but also difficulty in softcopy interpretation, including comparisons with multiple previous studies, especially films, and costs. It would seem that none of these are insurmountable.

Etta D. Pisano is a leader in digital mammography research and in evaluation of its clinical applications. She is the Principle Investigator for the ACRIN (American College of Radiology Imaging Network) Digital Mammography Imaging Screening Trial (DMIST). She is a Professor of Radiology and Biomedical Engineering at the University of North Carolina School of Medicine and has been Chief of Breast Imaging at UNC-Lineberger Comprehensive Cancer Center since 1989. She is one of my favorite people, a wise woman, with much to teach on this topic!

Dr. Pisano has assembled a group of recognized and experienced authorities, including Martin J. Yaffe, PhD, Professor of Medical Imaging and Medical Biophysics at the University of Toronto, Robert M. Nishikawa, PhD, Professor of Radiology at the University of Chicago, Fred M. Behlen, PhD, of LAI Technology, and Cherie M. Kuzmiak, DO, Assistant Professor of Radiology at the University of North Carolina School of Medicine, and UNC-Lineberger Comprehensive Cancer Center. The first three are old-timers and world-renowned experts in their fields. Cherie is a rising star in evaluating the clinical, educational, and research applications of digital mammography.

This group has produced a comprehensive review and update on digital mammography. Digital Mammography is a very useful book for anyone doing breast imaging, whether a breast imaging subspecialist or a general radiologist. It will also serve as an excellent reference source for anyone interested in the subject. Digital mammography is here to stay, and this is a very valuable source of information on it.

In short, these experts have put together a terrific resource on a complex topic! Enjoy!

Robert McLelland, MD, FACR
Clinical Professor, Department of Radiology
University of North Carolina School of Medicine
Chapel Hill, North Carolina
March 6, 2003

PREFACE

The first digital mammography unit, the General Electric Senographe 2000 D, was approved for sale in the United States in February 2000, with two other units approved by Spring, 2002. A very large number of digital mammography units have now been installed worldwide. In addition, several other companies are preparing Food and Drug Administration (FDA)-approval applications for their own devices. Recently, the U.S. Congress passed legislation authorizing increased Medicare reimbursement for this new technology over the traditional screen-film mammography. The number of radiologists and technologists who will be exposed to this technology and who will want to perform and interpret digital mammograms as part of their practices is expected to increase dramatically over the next 5 to 10 years, as more practices acquire the technology and more patients request it. Many physicists will be needed to assume responsibility for overseeing the quality control programs for this technology.

The technology has reached a level of maturity that motivated the writing of this book. Many cases have now demonstrated pathology that can be used for illustrative purposes. In addition, a great deal of information is available that details how the technology performed in clinical trials. Although some of the upcoming extra features are still under development, enough preliminary information is available to describe in detail how they will most likely fit into clinical practice once they are available.

The information in this book details everything that is currently known about the technology. This includes discussions about the basic advantages and disadvantages of the technology as compared to traditional screen-film mammography, technical descriptions of the available detector technologies and what advances are likely in the next few years, and the quality control programs that are most likely to be implemented under the U.S. Mammography Quality Standards Act (MQSA).

Aside from these technical details, this book analyzes the clinical trials on digital mammography performed to date. The studies compare digital mammography to screen-film mammography in both screening and diagnosis, and evaluates the various image processing algorithms that have been applied to digital mammography.

In addition, the book includes a thorough description of how this new technology interfaces with the new all-digital departments that are becoming the standard in modern radiology practices. This level of detail is provided in the chapter contributed by Fred Behlen, PhD, on PACS issues. Even those who are experienced with digital data handling will find this information extremely useful. The sheer size of the images, both in terms of pixel size and bit depth, requires special consideration and attention from those interested in maintaining data archives containing digital mammograms. This chapter will serve as a primer regarding such issues as they pertain to modern radiology practice.

No book on digital mammography would be complete without a thorough description of what the future holds and what tools will become available in the near future to improve its diagnostic accuracy. Therefore, this book provides detailed descriptions of computer-aided diagnosis and detection, image processing, tomosynthesis, and digital subtraction mammography. In addition, the expected advances in softcopy display for digital mammography, with implementation of some of these advanced applications, are discussed. Anyone who wants a glimpse into the future will enjoy these chapters.

Finally, the book ends with a complete atlas of digital mammography cases, with virtually every type of mammographic lesion demonstrated, including the appropriate work-up images and pathologic diagnoses. Radiologists and technologists taking care of patients and planning the transition to the use of digital mammography will appreciate the exhaustive detail included in these chapters.

We believe everything is here that anybody currently working with digital mammography needs to know to optimize his or her practice and use this new technology to maximum advantage. We hope that radiologists, physicists, and others will gain as much reading it as we have learned by writing it !

Etta D. Pisano, MD, FACR
Professor of Radiology and Biomedical Engineering
Department of Radiology
University of North Carolina School of Medicine
UNC-Lineberger Comprehensive Cancer Center
Chapel Hill, North Carolina

ACKNOWLEDGMENTS

Etta D. Pisano would like to extend special thanks to her husband, Jan Kylstra, and her children, Carolyn, Jim, Schuyler and Marijke, for their tremendous patience, tolerance, and unending support throughout the creation of this book. Special thanks for their extra support and encouragement over the years go to her two special professional mentors, Robert McLelland and Ferris Hall. Finally, Marcia Koomen, Dag Pavic, Ann Sherman, Jason Hauser, Beverly Currence, Yuanshui Zheng, Marylee Brown, Joseph K.T. Lee, Cathreen Gitia, Meghan Childers, and Natalie Harvey kept the other activities of work and home going at full speed throughout her work on this book. Without their support and extra work, she could not have set aside the time needed to complete this project.

Cherie M. Kuzmiak would like to thank Fumiko Tessien-Reading, MD, of the Department of Pathology at the University of North Carolina at Chapel Hill for the histology images. In addition, she would like to express her gratitude to Tanya Sherin and her staff at the Department of Medical Illustration at the University of North Carolina at Chapel Hill for their outstanding work. Finally, she would also like to thank Stacy Kuzmiak for many hours of support during this project.

Martin J. Yaffe is grateful for the scientific inspiration and constructive criticism provided over the years by his friend and colleague, Don Plewes, MD, and for the clinical insights and deep commitment to breast imaging that have come from his collaborator, Roberta Jong, MD. Without the irrepressible enthusiasm and amazing technical skills of Gordon Mawdsley, he would not have even considered attempting many projects, since Mr. Mawdsley was key to their success. Dr. Yaffe is also indebted to his graduate students and laboratory members who have done much of the work and developed many of the ideas described in his chapters. Finally, his wife, Robin Alter, has been a constant source of support, encouragement, humor, and energy through the ups and downs of the development of digital mammography. She truly operates on a higher plane.

DIGITAL MAMMOGRAPHY

1

CLINICAL DIGITAL MAMMOGRAPHY: OVERVIEW AND INTRODUCTION

Breast imaging has changed dramatically over the last two decades. Mammography's role as the most important tool for the early detection of breast cancer has become more universally accepted. This has been facilitated by improvements in the technology itself (1), as well as by the implementation of U.S. federal regulations governing quality assurance practices (2).

Technological improvements included the development of dedicated mammography equipment, the selection and use of appropriate tube and target material, added beam filtration, and the use of lower kilovolt-peak setting. These all improved image contrast. The widespread use of radiographic grids and improved compression paddles lessened the scatter radiation that degraded image quality. Shortened exposure times and smaller focal spot sizes reduced image blur. The widespread use of automatic exposure control provided optimal optical density for proper viewbox interpretation of mammograms (1). In addition, the more frequent use of geometric magnification provided improved detail for lesions that had been detected at screening (3) and allowed for more judicious decision-making regarding the need for breast biopsy (4). At the same time, dedicated high contrast film-screen products were developed, with an emphasis on tailoring film processing to the needs of the individual products being used in each clinic (5).

Of course, the improvements in image quality itself were made more universally available in the United States after the passage and implementation of the federal Mammography Quality Standards Act (MQSA) in 1992. This legislation created a statutory requirement for sites to meet what had been voluntary quality standards under the American College of Radiology (ACR) Mammography Accreditation Program (MAP) (6). The regulations, implemented by the U.S. Food and Drug Administration (FDA), provided ongoing experience and continuing education standards for interpreting physicians, medical physicists, and mammography technologists, as well as detailed requirements for ongoing documentation of equipment performance assessment. In addition, the regulations required annual on-site inspection of all mammography facilities, as well as clinical and phantom image review by an accrediting body every three years. Under the burden of this legislation, mammography facilities were forced to meet high standards in the performance of an admittedly imperfect test (7), the only one that has repeatedly been demonstrated to reduce breast cancer mortality.

Still, the value of screening mammography is not universally accepted even today (8), especially for women younger than 50 years of age (9). The National Institutes of Health (NIH) Consensus Panel Report of 1997 concluded that the reduction in mortality attributable to screening mammography was approximately 30% for women over 50 years of age, but might only reach 18% for women between the ages of 40 and 50 (10). This finding may be partially the result of the more aggressive natural history of breast cancer in younger women, when early detection may not offer a survival benefit for the majority of lesions detected (11). In addition, younger women are more likely to have radiographically dense breasts, and mammography has been shown to be less sensitive when breast tissue is more difficult to penetrate (12). Interestingly, radiographic density has been shown to correlate positively with risk (13), suggesting that the screening modality of choice is least sensitive in precisely those women who have the greatest risk. As a result, some experts have advocated that women receive different recommendations based on their individual risk profiles, particularly for younger women (14).

In fact, the sensitivity of screening with screen-film mammography is far from perfect, with many palpable or sonographically evident lesions not detectable by mammography (15,16). Published sensitivities have ranged from 45% to 88% (17). In addition, even when breast cancer is discovered on a screening mammogram, evidence may show that it has been present, but not visible, for up to five years previously (18)! Because earlier detection might yield an even greater number of cures, screening tools need to be improved so that breast cancer might be visible as soon as it exists in the breast.

Furthermore, some data suggest that screening mammography is also less specific in younger women. One prominent study suggests that the risk of a false–positive study to an individual patient who begins screening at age 40 is 50% (19). This is undoubtedly the result of the high incidence of noncancerous conditions, such as fibrocystic change and fibroadenomas in the breasts of perimenopausal women (20). In fact, the published rate of positive screening mammograms in a screening population in the United States ranges from 1.9% to 15%, depending primarily on the expertise of the reader and the presence of old films for comparison (21,22). Of course, most of these callbacks for an additional workup after screening mammograms are false–positives, given that the rate of breast cancer in a screening population varies from 4 to 7 per thousand.

It was in this context of insufficiently high sensitivity and specificity, with many experts highly critical of the efficacy of screening mammography in reducing breast cancer mortality (17), that the NIH convened an expert panel in 1991 (23). The panel addressed the question of where to invest research dollars for technology development. The attendees compared the desirability of further investments in the contemporary standard, screen-film mammography versus the development of a new technology, digital mammography. The group voted overwhelmingly in favor of digital mammography.

With that hallmark recommendation, the race was on. With NIH financial support and encouragement, many companies and research labs began the long process from design to development and clinical testing of digital mammography. This culminated in FDA approval of the first digital mammography system in the year 2000.

Why was the decision to develop digital mammography so evident to the experts consulted by the NIH in September 1991? The apparent advantages of digital technology are straightforward and self-evident to anyone who has ever used a digital camera. Digital images are more easily stored and retrieved than film images. Experts connected on-line around the world can view and offer opinions of the images. The original data are more difficult to lose, because they can be copied numerous times without loss of data quality. It is easier to provide a high-quality image with fewer exposures because the raw data can be processed and manipulated to view areas of interest in the image, possibly reducing the need for reexposures. In addition, computer software programs can be developed to assist the radiologist in interpreting the digital data in the images, without the burden present in film mammography, in which the image must first be digitized. Furthermore, once mammography is digital, three-dimensional reconstructions, tomographic imaging, and dual-energy and contrast-subtraction imaging are all more readily achievable at a low dose. All of these advantages and potential advances will be discussed in detail in the chapters in this text. The experts on the NIH panel were also hoping that improved sensitivity and speci-

ficity might be achieved by the high-resolution detectors that were to be developed as part of this effort, potentially at a lower radiation dose than is required with the screen-film technology.

Despite the initial optimism, the road to FDA approval and the U.S. marketing of digital mammography products has not been without significant problems (23). The initial FDA guidelines for manufacturers required that the manufacturer show that the new equipment was equivalent to traditional mammography. This was done by demonstrating agreement among readers proposed by FDA to be viewing both sets of images, without regard to the true breast cancer status of the patients imaged. Unfortunately, these guidelines were flawed in that they required digital mammography to have a higher rate of interreader agreement with screen-film mammography than was achievable between readers of screen-film mammography alone (24). After at least one company completed a clinical trial based on these initially flawed recommendations, the FDA released new guidelines requiring receiver operator curve (ROC) statistical analysis, with reference to the patient's known breast cancer status. In addition, while the original guidelines allowed for the companies to submit a 510K FDA application, the new guidelines required the more expensive and less easily amended Pre-Market Approval (PMA).

Why was the FDA so careful when allowing this new technology on the market, despite its evident promise? It is likely that FDA officials, who were responsible for the approval of this technology before marketing, were extremely sensitive to its potential limitations as well as its presumed benefits. They were undoubtedly also cognizant of the high profile that mammography has in the eyes of insurers, healthcare consumers, and breast cancer advocates. They did not want to approve a technology and later learn that it provided less sensitive screening for low contrast, subtle breast cancers.

What technical features available with the new technology raise concerns about the potential sensitivity of this technology for the early diagnosis of breast cancer? As will be discussed in the chapters to follow, digital mammography has *lower* spatial resolution than the current standard, screen-film mammography. Despite the ability to access and manipulate the contrast in the image, this may mean that small lesions, such as clustered calcifications, may go undetected with this technology. In addition, the viewing of all the available information in the image, specifically all the contrast and full spatial resolution, is impossible when the images are printed to film and very challenging even with currently available softcopy display systems. That is, when an image is printed, the viewer must choose how the image should be displayed and that choice necessarily limits the available contrast to some fixed value. As shown in the atlas of digital mammography cases, breast cancer with digital mammography looks just like breast cancer with film mammography. But, making that breast cancer evident on the image requires selecting the appropriate version of the image from the multitude of versions potentially available. In addition, for most units, viewing the image at full size on softcopy display stations requires an interaction that makes all parts of the image visible at full spatial resolution. This function is called "roam and zoom." For the high-spatial resolutions required in mammography, even digital mammography, this is more complicated ergonomically than other ordinary Picture Archiving and Communication System (PACS) tasks. Such interaction with digital mammograms likely requires special training of readers, as is currently mandated under MQSA (6).

So, although digital mammography holds great promise, because of the differences between it and film mammography, it is important that digital mammography be submitted to rigorous evaluation through clinical trials. That way, it can be proven to be the technology most suitable for the detection of breast cancer and the diagnosis of lesions of the breast. A review of the available literature on the clinical accuracy of this technology for screening and diagnosis, including a review of the data submitted to FDA as part of the PMA process, will be included in Chapter 4.

Breast cancer mortality in the United States and the United Kingdom has been falling at least for the last decade (26). We certainly hope that this trend will be accelerated with the universal implementation of digital mammography. However, it is only after critical evaluation that radiologists should discard a well-proven technology, screen-film mammography, for one that is quite promising.

REFERENCES

1. Haus AG. Technologic improvements in screen-film mammography. Radiology. 1990;74:628–637.
2. Bassett LW. The regulation of mammography. Sem Ultrasound, CT, MRI 1996;17:415–423.
3. Sickles EA, Doi K, Genant HK. Magnification film mammography: Image quality and clinical studies. Radiology 1977;125:69–76.
4. Sickles EA. Periodic mammographic follow-up of probably benign lesions: results of 3,184 consecutive cases. Radiology 1991;179:463–468.
5. Haus AG. Recent advances in screen-film mammography. Radiol Clin North Am 1987;25:913–928.
6. FDA. Quality mammography standards: Final rule. Federal Register. 1997;62:852–994.
7. Monsees BS. The Mammography Quality Standards Act. An overview of the regulations and guidance. Radiol Clin North Am 2000;38:759–772.
8. Horton R. Screening mammography—an overview revisited. Lancet 2001;358:1284–1285.
9. Harris R, Leininger L. Clinical strategies for breast cancer screening: weighing and using the evidence. Ann Intern Med 1995;122:539–547.
10. NIH Consensus Statement. Breast cancer screening for women ages 40–49. NIH Consensus Statement. 1997;15:1–35.
11. Moskowitz M. Breast cancer: Age-specific growth rates and screening strategies. Radiology. 1986;161:37–41.
12. Saarenmaa I, Salminen T, Geiger U, et al. The effect of age and density of the breast on the sensitivity of breast cancer diagnostic by mammography and ultrasonography. Breast Cancer Res Treat 2000;67:117–123.
13. Byng JW, Yaffe MJ, Lockwood GA, et al. Automated analysis of mammographic densities and breast carcinoma risk. Cancer 1997;80:66–74.
14. Gail M, Rimer B. Risk-based recommendations for mammographic screening for women in their forties. J Clin Oncol 1998;16:3105–3114.
15. Durfee SM, Selland DL, Smith DN, et al. Sonographic evaluation of clinically palpable breast cancers invisible on mammography. Breast J 2000;6:247–251.
16. Kaplan SS. Clinical utility of bilateral whole-breast US in the evaluation of women with dense breast tissue. Radiology 2001;221:641–649.
17. Fletcher SW, Black W, Harris R, et al. Report on the International Workshop on Screening for Breast Cancer. J Natl Cancer Inst 1993;85:1644–1656.
18. Spratt JS, Meyer JS, Spratt JA. Rates of growth of human neoplasms. Part II. J Surg Oncol 1996;61:68–83.
19. Elmore JG, Barton MB, Moceri VM, et al. Ten-year risk of false positive screening mammograms and clinical breast examinations. N Engl J Med 1998;338:1089–1096.
20. Love SM, Gelman RS, Silen W. Sounding board. Fibrocystic "disease" of the breast—a nondisease? N Engl J Med 1982;307:1010–1014.
21. Yankaskas BC, Cleveland RJ, Schell MJ, et al. Association of recall rates with sensitivity and positive predictive values of screening mammography. AJR 2001;177:543–549.
22. Bird RE. Professional quality assurance for mammography screening programs. Radiology 1990;177:587–590.
23. Shtern F. Digital mammography and related technologies: A perspective from the National Cancer Institute. Radiology 1992;183:629–630.
24. Pisano ED. Current status of full-field digital mammography. Radiology 2000;214:26–28.
25. Pisano ED, Braeuning MP, Chakraborty D, et al. An open letter to our congressmen and senators on digital mammography. Diagn Imag 1999;21:33–34.
26. Peto R, Boreham J, Clarke M, Davies C, et al. UK and USA breast cancer deaths down 25% in year 2000 at ages 20–69 years. Lancet 2000;355:1822–1825.

PHYSICS OF DIGITAL MAMMOGRAPHY

MARTIN J. YAFFE

The goal of mammography is to provide contrast between a lesion that is possibly residing within the breast and the normal surrounding tissue. Figure 2-1 illustrates a simple physicist's model of the breast, incorporating several key features for imaging. The breast varies in thickness and contains structures with different x-ray attenuation properties. Contrast arises from differences in x-ray transmission that are related to differences in tissue composition.

X-rays are attenuated exponentially as they pass through tissue or any other material, so that the number transmitted by the breast is given by the following formula, $n = n_0 \, e^{-\mu z}$, where n_0 is the number of x-rays incident on the breast, z is its thickness and μ is the x-ray attenuation coefficient of the tissue. One of the challenges of mammography arises from the similarity in the x-ray attenuation coefficients of normal breast tissue and cancer (Fig. 2-2). This causes differences in transmission to be very small. As illustrated in Figure 2–3, the inherent contrast for both tumors and microcalcifications falls as the energy increases. To maximize contrast, low-energy x-ray beams are commonly used in screen-film mammography. In addition, it is important that the imag-ing system be capable of recording the signal that results from transmitted x-rays very precisely.

COMPARISON OF CONVENTION AND DIGITAL MAMMOGRAPHY

Limitations of Conventional Mammography

In conventional screen-film mammography, x-rays are absorbed by a fluorescent screen, and the emitted light is recorded on photographic film to form the image. Although in many cases the performance of conventional mammography is excellent, this technical approach has several limitations, which if overcome, might lead to improved sensitivity of breast cancer detection and more accurate radiological diagnosis. Some of these limitations are:

1. Nonlinearity and saturation of the response of the film.
2. Inability to adjust brightness and contrast on the film image.

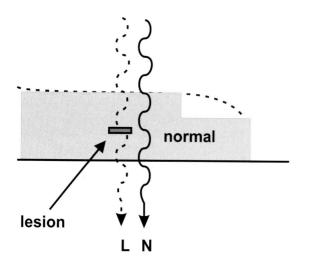

FIGURE 2-1. A schematic diagram of the breast illustrating the basic imaging problem of detecting differences in x-ray transmission between the lesion and normal tissue in a breast of varying thickness.

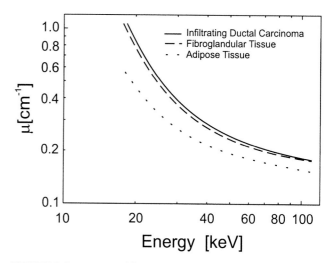

FIGURE 2-2. Measured linear x-ray attenuation coefficients of fat, fibroglandular tissue, and tumor in the breast. (From Johns and Yaffe (6).)

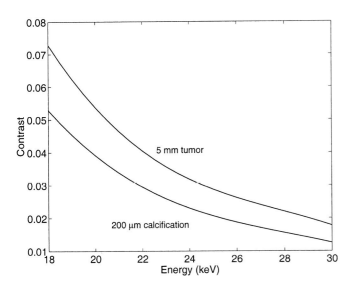

FIGURE 2-3. Dependence on contrast of a breast mass and a calcification on x-ray energy. In this example, the breast is 5 cm thick and composed of 50% fat and 50% fibroglandular tissue. The tumor is modeled as being cubic: 5 mm thick, 5 mm on a side. The calcification is a 0.2 mm cube.

3. Incomplete absorption of x-rays by the fluorescent screen—quantum noise.
4. Granularity of the film emulsion.
5. Scattered radiation.

Film Response

In screen-film mammography, the relationship between the x-rays transmitted by the breast and the optical density of the displayed image is highly nonlinear, as shown in Figure 2-4. Note that where the x-ray intensity is low, there is very little change of optical density on the processed film with change in x-ray intensity. This also occurs at high intensities, where there is almost no increase in blackness on the

already very dark film. The optical density "saturates" because all of the available silver in the film emulsion has already been used to form the image. This behavior, which is characteristic of film, causes the display contrast of the mammogram to be reduced. The display contrast is a result of the gradient or slope of the characteristic curve of the film. Where this is large, a small subject contrast (relative difference x-rays interacting with the screen) gives rise to an appreciable change in optical density of the developed film. The gradient of a mammographic film is illustrated in Figure 2-5. This was obtained by calculating the slope of the curve of Figure 2–4. It is seen that the gradient is reduced for both low and high x-ray intensities (i.e., in regions where the breast is relatively opaque and also where it is thinner or fatty and, therefore, relatively lucent).

If a film with a higher maximum gradient is chosen, the range of exposures over which relatively high gradients are available (known as the exposure latitude) is reduced. Conversely, films with increased latitude can be purchased, but normally only with a reduction in display gradient. One way of avoiding this problem to some extent is to produce film with very high maximum optical density. This allows improved latitude with high gradient, but necessitates viewing the film with extremely high brightness illuminators. This imposes viewing problems if there are bright areas on the film or if the edges of the films are not well masked. The reason is that the eye can be dazzled by the unattenuated light, deteriorating its contrast sensitivity.

Fixed Display Characteristics

The problem with the shape of the characteristic curve is compounded by the fact that once the film has been processed, it is not possible to alter its display characteristics. Therefore, even though some information may have been recorded on the film, it may not be displayed optimally to the radiologist. If the contrast on a screen-film mammogram is not adequate, the only way to improve the image is to

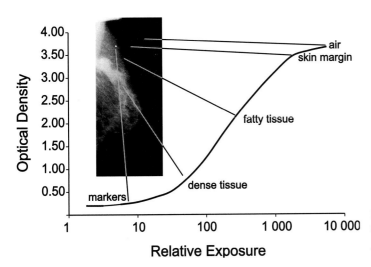

FIGURE 2-4. Characteristic (H&D) curve of a mammographic screen-film system. Optical density (OD) of the processed film is plotted versus the log of the relative x-ray exposure to the fluorescent screen.

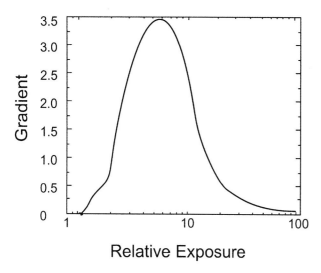

FIGURE 2-5. Gradient of the characteristic curve indicates the amount of contrast enhancement (or diminution) provided by the film as a display device. The range of exposures over which the gradient is near its maximum value provides a measure of the display latitude or dynamic range.

acquire another mammogram. This exposes the patient to additional radiation and is time consuming and costly.

Quantum Noise

X-rays are absorbed in a random manner following the Poisson statistical distribution. That means that even for a part of the breast whose x-ray attenuation was absolutely constant, if the average number of x-rays recorded per unit area was $\langle n \rangle$ this number would fluctuate from location to location with a standard deviation of $\sigma = \sqrt{\langle n \rangle}$. This fluctuation, which has nothing to do with variations in the breast, is known as quantum noise, or mottle. The relative quantum fluctuation (σ divided by the average) is then $\sqrt{\langle n \rangle}/\langle n \rangle$ or simply $1/\sqrt{\langle n \rangle}$, that is, the relative fluctuation or apparent noise in an x-ray image is inversely proportional to the square root of the amount of radiation absorbed by the detector. Alternatively, we can define the signal-to-noise ratio (SNR) as the inverse of the relative fluctuation, in this case as $\langle n \rangle/\sigma = \sqrt{\langle n \rangle}$. Therefore, if it is desired to reduce the apparent noisiness of the image (i.e., increase the SNR) to allow the perception of more subtle features, the radiation level absorbed by the screen should be increased. This can be accomplished in two ways: by increasing the exposure factors (i.e., mAs) or by employing a screen with a higher quantum interaction efficiency, η. The quantum interaction efficiency is simply the fraction of the x-rays falling on the image receptor that interacts with it. In screen-film imaging, each of these approaches has important difficulties.

The first is related to the shape of the characteristic curve of the film (Fig. 2-4). As a result of increase in exposure to the screen, parts of the image that would normally be recorded in the high gradient region of the characteristic curve of the film, might be recorded in the relatively flat "shoulder," where contrast would be diminished. Thus, an attempt to improve the image quality by reducing noise might actually result in a degradation of image quality.

Second, a well-known property of screen-film radiography is that the spatial resolution of the image deteriorates as the fluorescent screen becomes thicker. This effect is illustrated in Figure 2-6, which compares thick and thin screens. When the x-ray is absorbed, light is produced and the light quanta diverge from their point of creation. The thicker the screen, the more spreading occurs before the light can reach the surface of the screen and be collected. This is characterized by the line-spread function, which describes the spatial distribution of the light collected when the screen is irradiated by a narrow line of x-rays. The greater lateral spread of light in a thick screen causes the line-spread function of a thick screen to be wider (poorer resolution) than for a thinner screen. Therefore, if it is necessary, as in mammography, to have high spatial resolution, then the phosphor screen must be made relatively thin. This limits the value of η, causing many of the incident x-rays to pass through the screen without interaction. The implications of wasting of x-rays are twofold: fewer x-rays contribute to the image and therefore the relative noise is higher and, because it is necessary to make up for the lost x-rays in order to obtain a target optical density, the dose received by the breast is higher than that ideally required.

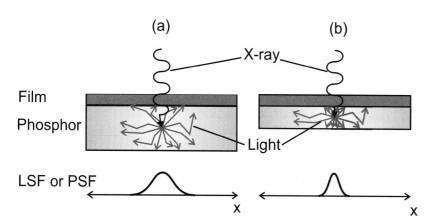

FIGURE 2-6. Schematic showing the production of light at an x-ray interaction site in a phosphor and the spreading of the light quanta as they move toward the collection surface. **(a)** thick phosphor, **(b)** thinner phosphor.

Film Granularity

Photographic film has a granular structure that becomes very obvious under magnification. This graininess, which is random, imposes a fluctuation, or noise, on the image in addition to the quantum noise. This increases the relative fluctuation above the level determined by the number of quanta used and reduces the SNR.

Scattered Radiation

In mammography, some x-rays will pass through the breast without interaction; some will be absorbed; and some will scatter in the breast and escape. Of the scattered x-rays, some will be directed toward the imaging system. At mammographic energies for an average breast, the number of these per unit area may be on the order of 70% as many as the number of directly transmitted rays (1,2). Recording of scattered x-rays has several effects on a screen-film mammogram. First, part of the useful range of the film is taken up by recording scattered radiation, which is not considered to carry useful information. Second, a fairly uniform haze is imposed over the entire image. Finally, recording the scatter adds statistical fluctuation without information, thereby reducing the SNR.

In screen-film mammography, scatter directed toward the image receptor is partially removed by an antiscatter grid. The grid is not efficient, in that it removes part (25%–30%) of the useful directly transmitted "primary" x-ray beam, while rejecting most, but not all (80%–90%), of the scattered radiation (3,4). The loss of both primary and scattered radiation reduces the number of x-rays recorded by the receptor, and in film this must be replaced by increased exposure from the x-ray tube to ensure that the film is exposed to the proper level on its characteristic curve. The required increase in the tube output (and the radiation dose to the breast) is called the Bucky factor, and it can be on the order of 2–2.5.

Characterizing Imaging Performance

To evaluate imaging systems or to compare the performance of a novel system to a conventional imaging device, it is necessary to have performance measures. Important imaging parameters to be considered are spatial resolution, contrast, noise characteristics, and dynamic range. Some elements, such as SNR have already been mentioned. Others will be discussed below.

Modulation Transfer Function

Spatial resolution can be assessed by determining the limiting resolution in terms of line-pairs/mm from a bar pattern. This is a subjective test, however, that is not very useful in the analysis of complex imaging systems.

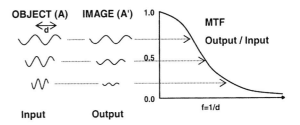

FIGURE 2-7. Illustrating the concept of modulation transfer function (MTF). Sinusoidal transmission patterns of different spatial frequencies, but constant amplitude are imaged and the output amplitude is compared to that of the input at each frequency.

A preferable measurement is the modulation transfer function (MTF). The MTF (Fig. 2-7) describes how well the imaging system or a device within it, such as an image receptor, transfers the contrast of simple shapes (sinusoidal patterns) from the incident x-ray pattern to the output. A sinusoid is a repetitive function, characterized by having a frequency and an amplitude. In this case, the frequency is a spatial frequency in cycles/mm. The concept of spatial frequency can be visualized by considering ripples in a pond. Low spatial frequencies (long distance between wave peaks) represent coarse structures, and high spatial frequencies (short wavelengths) describe fine detail.

Any pattern can be represented as a collection or recipe of sinusoidal shapes, each spatial frequency having a specific amplitude. If one knows how each spatial frequency is transferred through a system, then the performance of the system at imaging the object or pattern is known. The MTF of an imaging system is often 1.0 at very low spatial frequencies and falls with increasing spatial frequency. An important feature of the MTF is that in systems containing several factors affecting spatial resolution, the overall MTF is determined as the product of the MTFs of the individual components. For example, the MTF of a radiographic system is the product of that due to the focal spot, the detector, and any motion of the patient during the exposure. This is helpful in determining what part of the system is responsible for limiting its performance. The MTF of a typical screen-film system is shown in Figure 2-8. As seen from the figure, it extends well beyond 20 cycles/mm. It is mainly determined by the screen, as the film has a very high MTF.

Detective Quantum Efficiency

The SNR is an effective quantitative description of the quality of the information carried by the radiological image. The bigger the signal is compared to the random fluctuation, the better the image is. As discussed above, SNR increases with increasing exposure and with higher values of η. It is decreased when there are sources of noise other than quantum noise contributing to the image. We can think of the highest SNR as that carried by the x-rays leaving the

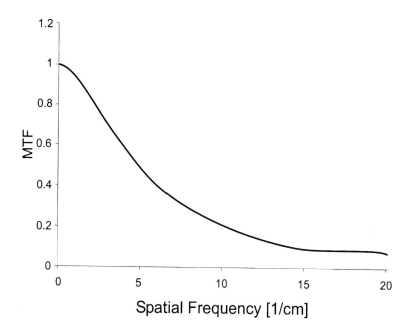

FIGURE 2-8. MTF of a modern screen-film system. (After Bunch (7)).

breast. If the number of x-ray quanta in a specified area were n_0, its value would be: $SNR_{in} = \langle n_o \rangle / \sqrt{\langle n_o \rangle} = \sqrt{\langle n_o \rangle}$.

For a system that was perfect except that the detector did not absorb all incident x-rays, the signal would be $\eta \langle n_o \rangle$ and the noise $\sqrt{\eta \langle n_o \rangle}$, giving a reduced SNR of $\sqrt{\eta \langle n_o \rangle}$.

If SNR is a measure of the quality of the information in the image, the performance of the imaging system can be characterized by asking how well it transfers the input SNR to the system output (i.e., the observer). The detective quantum efficiency (DQE) measures this by computing $DQE = SNR^2_{out}/SNR^2_{in}$. For a perfect system, DQE would equal 1.0. Considering just the efficiency of x-ray interaction described above, DQE would be $\eta \langle n_o \rangle / n_o = \eta$. So the DQE would be just the quantum interaction efficiency, the fraction of incident x-rays used by the detector.

If other sources of noise are present, SNR_{out} will decrease below the value predicted by the number of interacting quanta, so that DQE will fall below η. From the measure-

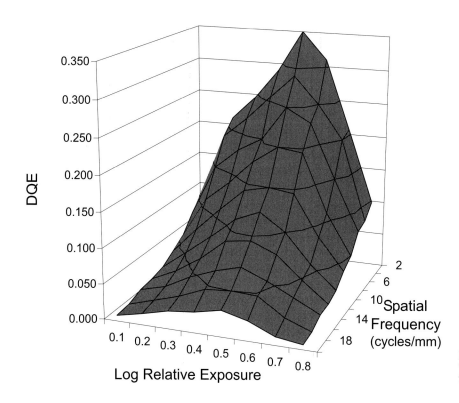

FIGURE 2-9. DQE versus spatial frequency for a mammographic screen-film combination. (Bunch (7)).

ment of SNR$_{out}$ it will appear that fewer x-rays have been used to form the image than has actually been the case, and DQE is a measure of that apparent lack of efficiency.

When DQE values are presented, they are usually given as a function of spatial frequency (5). DQE(f) tells at each level of detail how well the system transfers the SNR information present at its input. Figure 2-9 gives DQE results for a high-quality screen-film combination. Note that DQE for the mammographic screen-film system is, at best, approximately 45% and falls with increasing spatial frequency. It also has a maximum value at an intermediate x-ray intensity and falls for both lower and higher exposures. An ideal system for mammography would have a DQE of 100% at all spatial frequencies and x-ray intensities, as this implies production of an image with the most information for the amount of radiation dose received.

Digital Mammography

In digital mammography, the screen-film system is replaced by a detector, which produces an electronic signal that is digitized and stored. This effectively decouples the processes of image acquisition, storage, processing, and display, which in screen-film mammography are all intimately associated with the properties of the film. Whereas compromises must be made in screen-film mammography, for example between η and spatial resolution and between image contrast and exposure latitude, it should be possible to optimize each process in digital mammography.

Digital Image acquisition

The characteristic curve of a detector used for digital mammography is shown in Figure 2-10. The detector is designed to provide a signal which is highly linear (or logarithmic)

with radiation intensity and where the response does not flatten out at low or high intensities.

Acquisition of analog images, such as with film and digital images, are compared in Figure 2-11. In screen-film imaging, the image is more or less continuously defined in space and in optical density. For example, one can consider the value of OD at a position 3.5 cm from the left edge of the image or at 3.51 cm or even at 3.501 cm. While at some point the blurriness of the image makes this ridiculous, it can still, in principle, be done. Similarly, the OD can be measured and variations between 1.7, 1.75, and 1.755, and so on, could be recorded. Again, the noise in the image would eventually make this specification of precision futile. Digital images are sampled images. As illustrated in Figure 2-11b, signal measurements are only acquired and specified over a matrix of discrete image elements. These are defined by the size of the detector element, or del. Each element has a finite size, and the value assigned to it represents the average signal falling over its area. It is not possible to describe the image with finer spatial resolution than that of a del.

Similarly, the signal level is assigned one of a finite set of values ranging from 0 to 2^n-1, where n is the number of bits of digitization. The precision of image recording is determined in part by the number of bits. For example, a 12-bit system represents signal levels from 0 to 4,095. In such a system, if the actual signal presented by the detector corresponded, for example, to 1,203.5, it would be repre-

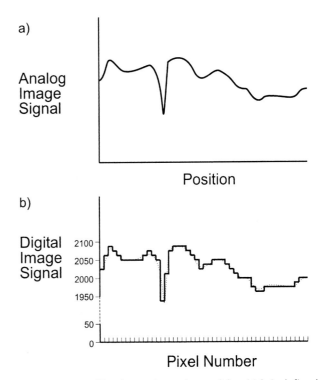

FIGURE 2-11. Unlike the analogue image **(a)**, which is defined continuously in space and signal level, the digital image **(b)** is pixelated at discrete points and only a finite number of signal levels are recorded.

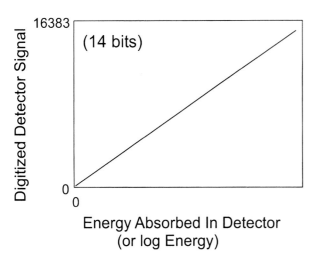

FIGURE 2-10. Characteristic curve for a digital mammography detector. Response is highly linear with x-ray input.

sented as either 1,203 or 1,204, because 1,203.5 does not exist. To gain such precision, a 13-bit system would be required, in which case, the signal would appear as 2,407 on a scale from 0 to 8,191.

Another difference between analog and digital mammography relates to image noise. As in screen-film imaging, image fluctuation is determined both by the number of x-rays that strike the detector (known as the quantum fluctuation or quantum mottle) and also the inherent granularity of the detector. In screen-film mammography, the film itself has a granular structure, which is unique to each sheet of film and, therefore, cannot be removed from the image. In most digital mammography systems, the same detector is used repeatedly. Therefore, any structure noise can be recorded and used as a "correction mask" to remove the effect of this "fixed pattern noise" from subsequent images.

Image Display

In digital mammography, the image data are displayed over a set of discrete picture elements (pixels), using either a printed film (hard copy) or a monitor (soft copy). When the images are displayed on a monitor, it is possible to interactively adjust not only the brightness and contrast but also the sharpness of the image. By using different display algorithms, or look-up tables (LUTs), the image can be displayed with arbitrary contrast and is not limited by the characteristic curve of the film. In addition, this processing allows the contrast of the displayed image to be independent of the basic x-ray subject contrast values given in Figure 2-3. Image display will be discussed in greater detail in Chapter 8.

PROPERTIES OF DIGITAL IMAGES

Spatial Resolution

The spatial resolution of the acquired digital image is determined by several factors, including the size of the del, the effective x-ray focal spot size and magnification, spread of signal in the detector, and relative motion among the x-ray source, breast, and detector. The effect of each factor can be described by a modulation transfer function (MTF) and the overall MTF determined as the product of the MTFs of the individual processes. In addition, the displayed spatial resolution can be further affected by the pixel (the size of the element actually used to display the image) size. The size of the pixel referenced to the breast can be larger (averaging), smaller (zooming), or the same as that of the del.

Del Size

Most detectors are constructed as a set of discrete dels, as shown schematically in Figure 2-12. Each del has an active area with dimension, d, and this may be surrounded by an area that is insensitive to the incident radiation. This causes the pitch or spacing between dels, p, to be greater than d. The relative area of sensitivity d^2/p^2 is called the fill factor and this, in part, determines the geometric radiation efficiency of the detector.

The del size also determines the basic spatial resolution associated with the del. Because information is "smeared" over d, the smaller d is, the less blurring results and therefore, the higher the spatial resolution. As shown in Figure 2-13, the MTF associated with the del falls to 0* at a spatial frequency of 1/d cycles/mm. A detector with 50 μm dels passes spatial frequencies of up to 20 cycles/mm.

The pitch is also important in affecting image quality. The spacing between samples determines whether information is lost between measurements. If this occurs, a phenomenon called aliasing can result. To avoid aliasing, the pitch of the detector must be less than $1/(2\ f_{max})$, where f_{max}

---

*Note that the MTF does rise again at frequencies beyond the first zero; however, the information may not be reliably depicted beyond this point. For example, between the first and second zero points, there is a reversal of contrast, so that structures which should be dark space appear light and vice versa.

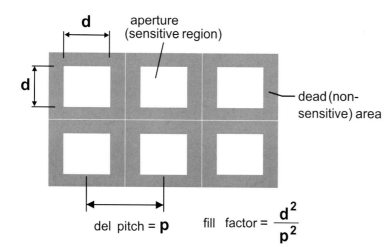

FIGURE 2-12. A detector element (del) contains an active region with dimension d. Dels are spaced at a pitch p. Because of inactive detector material on the del, the fraction of the area that is sensitive to x-rays, d^2/p^2, also known as the "fill factor," can be less than 1.

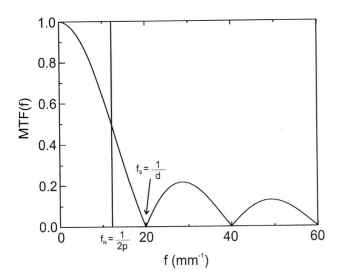

FIGURE 2-13. Theoretical MTF associated with a square del. The MTF reaches its first zero at a frequency of 1/d; however, frequencies above 1/2p are aliased, or misrepresented.

TABLE 2-1. FACTOR BY WHICH THE BREAST ATTENUATES INCIDENT X-RAYS VS. BREAST THICKNESS, COMPOSITION, AND ENERGY. CALCULATIONS ARE FOR MONOENERGETIC X-RAYS

Energy (keV)	Breast thickness (cm)	% Fibroglandular				
		0%	30%	50%	70%	100%
18	3	5	8	11	14	22
	4	9	16	24	35	61
	5	16	33	53	84	171
	6	28	66	117	205	477
	8	87	268	569	1,207	3,729
20	3	4	5	7	8	11
	4	6	9	12	16	25
	5	10	16	23	33	55
	6	15	29	44	66	123
	8	38	88	153	267	612
25	3	3	3	3	4	5
	4	4	5	5	6	8
	5	5	7	8	10	13
	6	7	10	12	15	21
	8	13	20	27	37	57
30	3	2	2	3	3	3
	4	3	3	4	4	5
	5	4	4	5	6	7
	6	5	6	7	8	10
	8	8	11	13	16	21

is the highest spatial frequency of information in the image. Otherwise, aliasing causes information at spatial frequencies greater than 1/(2p) to be represented at lower spatial frequency as illustrated in Figure 2-14. This not only misrepresents the higher spatial frequency information, but also interferes with the information that exists at the lower "aliased" frequency. Therefore, although 50 μm dels will pass information up to 20 cycles/mm, they only provide unaliased imaging up to 10 cycles/mm.

Dynamic Range (Latitude)

Both the range of intensities that can be recorded and also the level of precision are determined by the number of bits of digitization and the x-ray fluence (number of x-rays per unit area) incident on the breast. The imaging system

should have adequate range of response to accommodate the unattenuated x-ray beam at the edge of the breast without creating an artifact. At the same time, the system should be able to record with adequate precision the lowest signal level (i.e., that transmitted by the thickest and most attenuating region of the breast). The range of attenuations by breasts of different thicknesses and average compositions is illustrated in Table 2-1.

It is seen that for a thick breast (8 cm) that is highly dense (70% fibroglandular by volume), if an x-ray beam of

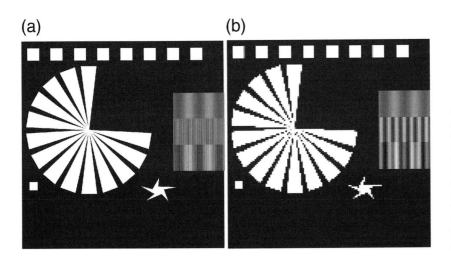

(a)　　　(b)

FIGURE 2-14. Illustrates aliasing. **(a)** Sinusoids at two frequencies, one below and one above $f_{max}/2$ are shown (*right side:* top and middle panels) as well as the combination of the two (lower panel). **(b)** If the sampling interval is too large, the higher frequency is not properly represented (middle panel) and appears as a lower frequency signal, interfering with the perception of the actual low frequency pattern in the combination (lower panel). These effects are also evident in the radial spoke and star objects.

effective energy 18 keV is used, the range of attenuation is about 1,207.

How Many Bits Are Required?

To cover the range of 1,207, a detector which had only about this range could be considered. Using the nearest number of bits encompassing that range, an 11-bit digitizer might be chosen. This would provide a range of 2,048 and would give ample precision for measuring small changes in attenuation in the breast in the thinnest regions where the signal level was high. But, when the full attenuation of 1,207 occurs, the signal from the digitizer will only be 2,047/1,207, which depending on the design of the digitizer would be "1" or "2." Clearly, it would be impossible to obtain any subtlety in image tone with such coarse digitization. If enough range of digitization is provided to allow 1% precision of measurement in the most attenuating part of the breast, a range of 1,207 × 100 = 120,700 would be required. This would require 17 bits (131,072 levels) of digitization. While this is conceivable, another approach that would definitely result in a lower dose to such a thick, dense breast and would require fewer bits of digitization, is to use a higher energy to acquire the image. For example, referring to Table 2-1, with an effective energy of 25 keV, the attenuation factor for the same breast would only be 37. Adjustment of the beam energy is normally done in digital mammography to control the required dynamic range and dose.

As an example, consider a breast that is 6-cm thick, composed primarily of fat, but with 3 cm of fibroglandular tissue in one area, as seen in Figure 2-15. If this is imaged at 20 keV, from Table 2-1, the attenuation factor in the fatty region would be 15, while in the fibroglandular region, it

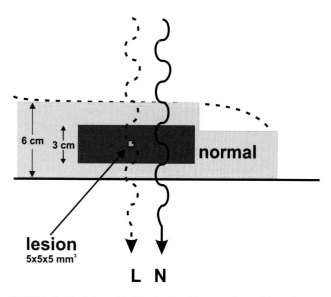

FIGURE 2-15. Schematic illustrating the problem of imaging a tumor in a dense part of the breast.

would be 44. For 1% precision, the range required would be 4,400. To obtain this precision, 12 bits would not quite be adequate (i.e., 13 bits would be required).

Now consider that the tumor modeled in Figure 2-3 is to be imaged. At 20 keV, the contrast of the tumor would be about 5.5%, so the precision of digitization would be adequate. In fact, on the basis of the number of bits, a tumor as thin as 1 mm could be imaged.

How Much Radiation Is Required?

In screen-film mammography, the number of x-rays that must be used to expose the breast is determined by the amount of energy that must be absorbed in the screen to give the required optical density in the processed film. In digital mammography, the exposure should be determined by the required SNR in the densest, thickest part of the breast.

In addition to an adequate number of bits of digitization, the actual radiation intensity recorded by the detector must be high enough to limit the relative x-ray fluctuation noise to an acceptable level and provide the necessary precision to detect subtle signal differences caused by lesions. For example, if 200 x-ray quanta were incident on a region of the detector corresponding to one image pixel and the detector had η = 50%, then, on average 100 x-rays would interact and the relative fluctuation in this value would be $1/(100)^{1/2}$ = 1/10 or 10%. Under these conditions, the SNR would be 10.

If instead, 20,000 x-rays (100 times more) were incident, the relative noise would be $1/(10,000)^{1/2}$ or 1%, that is, 10 times lower, and SNR would be 10 times higher. SNR scales with the square root of the number of interacting quanta.

Recall that to reduce the noise in an image, one can either expose the patient to more radiation or else use a detector with higher η. Conversely, if the detector has higher η, either the noise can be reduced without increasing dose or a dose reduction can be achieved without increase in noise.

To determine whether there are enough x-rays to detect a tumor in a certain background, compare the difference between the number of x-rays in the shadow of the tumor and in an equal area of surrounding tissue to the noise in that difference. This is called the signal-difference-to-noise-ratio, or SDNR. Now, considering the example of Figure 2-15, if a typical exposure yielding 1 Roentgen at the entrance to the breast were used, this would be reduced by a factor of 44 in passing through the dense part of the breast. Another factor of 3 might be lost because of the combination of the presence of the anti-scatter grid in the beam and the fact that η of the detector was less than 1. For a tumor, whose projected area in the image was 25 mm^2, the SDNR would be about 234, as illustrated in Figure 2-16A. Imaging theory suggests

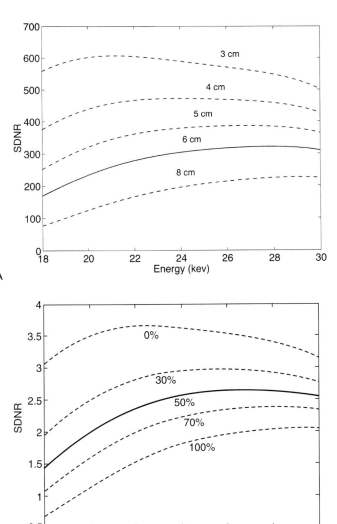

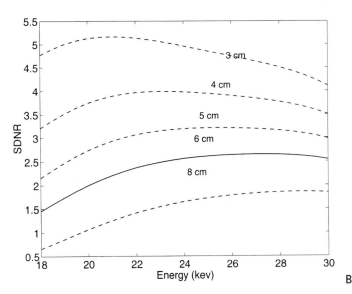

FIGURE 2-16. The signal difference to noise ratio (SDNR) determines whether a structure is statistically detectable in a noisy background. **(A)** For a breast whose composition is 50% fat/50% fibroglandular at the radiation doses used in current mammography, the SDNR is much more than adequate to detect masses. **(B)** For the same dose, the SDNR for microcalcifications may be near the point of limiting their detectability. **(C)** For denser breasts the SDNR falls even further.

that an SDNR of 5 would be adequate for reliable detection of the tumor. This suggests that much higher doses are being used than are theoretically necessary to perform this task. The tumor should be detectable with a dose reduction of $(234/5)^{1/2}$ or approximately a factor of 7 from the values used for screen-film mammography.

Such dose reduction is not acceptable for two reasons. First, the simple model of the tumor treats it as a cube, whereas, in reality, the contrast and signal difference would be greatly reduced at its edges where it was thinner. Second, we are also interested in detecting microcalcifications. While the contrast provided by a calcification as small as 200 microns is still reasonable (Fig. 2-3) because of the small area of the speck, the SDNR becomes so very small (Fig. 2-16B) that detection at this radiation level is marginal. The SDNR at a given radiation dose becomes further reduced for thicker breasts and for denser breasts (Fig. 2-16C), necessitating both an increase in effective energy used

for imaging and also an increase in the exposure used. Thus the radiation level required for digital mammography is largely determined by breast thickness, breast density, and the need to detect small calcifications. Because of the microcalcifications, except for improvements in the efficiency of the detector system or scatter rejection, the dose used in mammography should probably not be reduced much from current levels.

Energy Spectra for Digital Mammography

X-ray sources commercially available for mammography are not monoenergetic, but generally produce a spectrum similar to that shown in Figure 2-17. In screen-film mammography, the spectrum is chosen to provide the greatest practical contrast, while using an effective energy high enough such that the breast is reasonably well penetrated, and the dose is not excessive. This tends to drive the choice toward

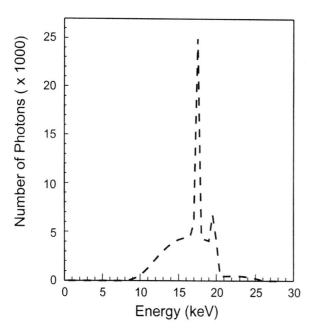

FIGURE 2-17. Spectrum for mammography x-ray source.

relatively low energies, for example, 26 kV with a molybdenum target x-ray tube and a molybdenum filter placed in the beam, as in Figure 2-17.

In digital mammography, the SDNR is more important than the contrast because contrast can always be increased in the display process. Figure 2-16 suggests that the SDNR does not change rapidly with energy, and the use of higher energies actually allows lower doses to be used and reduces the dynamic range requirements of the detector. As users become more familiar with digital mammography, they are departing more from exposure techniques that replicate those used with film and imaging with higher kilovoltage and with rhodium rather than molybdenum filtration in Mo target systems.

REFERENCES

1. Barnes GT, Brezovich IA. Contrast: effect of scattered radiation. In: Logan WW, ed. Breast Carcinoma: The Radiologist's Expanded Role. New York: Wiley, 1977;73–81.
2. Barnes GT, Brezovich IA. The intensity of scattered radiation in mammography. Radiology 1978;126:243–247.
3. Wagner, AJ. Contrast and grid performance in mammography. In: Barnes GT, Frey GD, eds. Screen-Film Mammography: Imaging Considerations and Medical Physics Responsibilities. Madison, WI: Medical Physics Publishing, 1991;115–134.
4. De Almeida A, Rezentes PS, Barnes GT. Mammography grid performance. Radiology 1999;210:227–232.
5. Bunch, PC, Huff, KE, Van Metter, R. Analysis of the detective quantum efficiency of a radiographic screen-film combination. J Opt Soc Am, 1987;A4:902–909.
6. Johns, PC, Yaffe, MJ. X-ray characterization of normal and neoplastic breast tissues. Phys Med Biol 1987;32:675–695.
7. Bunch, PC, The effects of reduced film granularity on mammographic image quality, in Medical Imaging 1997: Physics of Medical Imaging, R.Van Metter, J Beutel, Eds. Proc. SPIE 1997;3032: 302–317.

3

DETECTORS FOR DIGITAL MAMMOGRAPHY

MARTIN J. YAFFE
JAMES G. MAINPRIZE

Along with the image display system, the detector is one of the key elements of a digital mammography system. The role of the detector is to record the information carried by the pattern of x-rays transmitted by the breast. This should be done precisely and efficiently, over the entire range of intensities transmitted by different regions of the breast, without loss of information. The detector must provide the spatial resolution required for the examination. The stages of operation for a detector include the following,

1. Interaction with the x-rays transmitted by the breast.
2. Absorption of the energy carried by the x-rays.
3. Conversion of this energy to a usable signal—generally light or electrons.
4. Collection of this signal.
5. Secondary conversion (in the case of light).
6. Readout, amplification, and digitization.

To maximize imaging performance, all of these operations must be properly optimized. Detectors are characterized by their quantum interaction efficiency, sensitivity, spatial resolution properties, noise, dynamic range, and linearity of response.

QUANTUM INTERACTION EFFICIENCY

Quantum interaction efficiency, η, describes the fraction of the x-rays incident on the detector that interacts with it to produce some signal. The quantum interaction efficiency is given by the formula $\eta(E) = 1 - e^{-\mu(E)d}$ where $\mu(E)$ is the x-ray linear attenuation coefficient of the detector material, which depends on the x-ray energy, E, and d is the thickness of the detector. The quantum interaction efficiency increases with increasing d and η. The value of η depends on the density and atomic number of the absorber. Some linear attenuation coefficients are

given in Figure 3-1. In general, coefficients decrease as energy increases, causing η to do so as well. An exception occurs when the x-ray energy exceeds an absorption edge of the detector material. For example, as seen in Figure 3-1, at the K edge of iodine at 33 keV, the attenuation coefficient of CsI increases dramatically, providing improved η at energies above this point.

SENSITIVITY

Detector sensitivity is determined by several factors. These include: (1) η, (2) the fraction of the energy of the interacting quantum that is absorbed in the active detector material, (3) $1/w$, where w is the amount of energy required to produce an element of signal (a light quantum or an electron, whichever is being measured) and (d) the efficiency of collection and detection of the signal that is produced.

For material with relatively high atomic numbers (say, $Z > 30$) and for the low energies typically used in digital mammography (<50 keV), the majority of x-ray interactions in the detector are through the photoelectric effect and, therefore, most of the energy of the interacting x-ray is absorbed locally. For example, for the cesium in CsI(Tl) phosphor, more than 90% of interacting 30 keV x-rays are absorbed through the photoelectric effect; the remainder are scattered with a high probability of subsequent absorption. For incident x-rays above the K edge of the detector material, some of the energy will be reemitted as x-ray fluorescence, although again, it may be reabsorbed, particularly if careful attention is paid to detector design. This might involve the choice of specific detector materials for certain energies for imaging and appropriate combinations of elements in the detector, such that one absorbs the fluorescence produced by another.

The smaller the value of w, the greater the signal will be for a given number of interacting x-rays. Typical val-

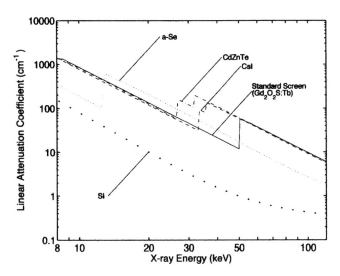

FIGURE 3-1. X-ray attenuation coefficients for common detector materials.

ues of *w* in electron volts are given in Table 3-1. For example, a 20 keV x-ray (20,000 eV) which interacts will produce 20,000/50 = 400 electron-hole pairs in a selenium detector. From Figure 3-1, a 0.1-mm thick Se detector will have η = 90% at 20 keV, so the sensitivity can be described by the statement that one incident x-ray will produce 360 e–h pairs.

NOISE

Ideally, the major source of random fluctuation in radiographic images is quantum noise. As discussed in Chapter 2, the effects of quantum noise can be controlled to achieve a desired SNR by detecting an adequate number of x-rays in each part of the image. This is accomplished by a combination of an adequate exposure to the patient, use of a beam of appropriate penetrating capability, so that enough quanta pass through the breast to strike the detector, and having as high a value of η for the detector as possible.

Although it is desirable for quantum noise to be the dominant cause of noise in an image, other possible noise sources must be considered, Optimization of system design involves controlling these noise sources.

TABLE 3-1. THE *W* VALUES FOR SOME DETECTOR MATERIALS

Material	*w* value (eV)
a-Se	50
PbI$_2$	4.8
CsI(Tl)	25
Gd$_2$O$_2$S:Tb	16

One form of noise is the structural fluctuation in sensitivity from del to del, sometimes referred to as fixed pattern noise. As discussed below, in most digital detector systems, to the extent that it is temporally constant, fixed pattern noise can be removed by a correction technique known as flat fielding. This correction is applied to each acquired image. The data used to establish the correction constants can be acquired as frequently as necessary according to the stability of the detector response.

Another source of fluctuation arises from the variation in the amount of secondary signal (e.g., number of light quanta produced by a phosphor) when an x-ray quantum interacts in the detector. This can arise from two sources. First, because there are competing mechanisms in the detector for energy absorption, a statistical distribution of signal is produced when an x-ray of fixed energy interacts. This phenomenon was studied by Swank and others (1). Expressions for the DQE of a detector include the product η A$_s$, where the Swank factor, A$_s$, describes the extent by which the DQE is reduced because of this effect. The second source of fluctuation of this type comes from the fact that the x-rays used for imaging are not monoenergetic, but instead are emitted in a spectrum, such as that shown in Figure 2-17 for a molybdenum target mammography tube. Each interacting x-ray carries a different amount of energy and, therefore, is expected to produce a different secondary signal. The effect on noise is statistically similar to that of the Swank effect and a similar factor can be used to describe its influence on the DQE.

The last noise source comes about when there are two stages of energy conversion—e.g., x-rays to light and then light to electrons as in systems employing a phosphor and photodetector. If the number of secondary signal quanta collected and detected per interacting x-ray is not much larger than 1, then we say that a "secondary quantum sink" exists. In this case, the statistical fluctuation in the detection of the secondary quanta becomes a significant noise source and may rival the primary quantum noise in importance. For this reason, it is important that the gain and collection efficiency of such systems be adequate. A classic example of a system where there is a secondary quantum sink is one in which a large-area phosphor is coupled by a demagnifying lens to a small-area optical recording system. Because of the inefficiency of the lens, only a small fraction of the light emitted from the screen is collected, giving rise to fluctuation in the measurement of the light.

DETECTOR CORRECTIONS

It is desirable that in the absence of spatial information in the breast, the image should be uniform. In screen-film technology, an enormous amount of effort is expended in making the components so that they have uniform response over their surface.

In a digital imaging system, it is often possible to correct for nonuniformities in sensitivity by performing a "flat-fielding" procedure. Consider two dels in the detector, each having slightly different linear responses, characterized by a dark signal (intercept) and a gain (slope) as illustrated in Figure 3-2a). First, a "dark" image is obtained by recording the detector response for the time equal to that of an x-ray exposure but without x-rays. This determines the "dark" values, D_1, D_2, and so on from all dels as shown in the inset to Figure 3-2a. The recorded value for each detector element, or del, is subsequently subtracted from each detector measurement thereby setting the corrected intercept from each del to zero. This measurement of the dark, or offset signal, can be updated as often as required (after every image if necessary) to correct for drifts in the detector offset values related to temperature variations as the system warms up or as the room temperature varies. There is still a difference in slopes or sensitivities of the dels as illustrated in Figure 3-2b.

Correction for variation in sensitivity simply involves exposing the detector to an x-ray beam that has passed through a uniform attenuator. The constant exposure, E_{cal}, received by all dels will produce different signals. This image is sometimes referred to as a correction mask. From these data, a correction constant can be determined for each del to give it the same apparent sensitivity as all the rest. For example, using this set of gain correction constants, the response of each del can be adjusted up or down to the average sensitivity of the detector.

During imaging, the acquired data from each del has its offset removed and then the remaining signal is divided by the corresponding gain correction constant to produce the corrected image. An example of this procedure is given in Figure 3-3 for both the image of a uniform attenuator and a mammogram. Note the dramatic improvement in uniformity of the image.

It is important to realize that like the image acquired from the breast, the mask used for flat-field correction will contain noise. Using the flat-fielding mask for correction will add noise to the resultant image. If the digital mammogram and the mask image were produced with the same amounts of radiation, the standard deviation of the image pixels would be increased by 2 (i.e., about 40%). To avoid unnecessary increase in image noise, it is important that the flat-field mask be produced using a much larger amount of radiation than used for each indi-

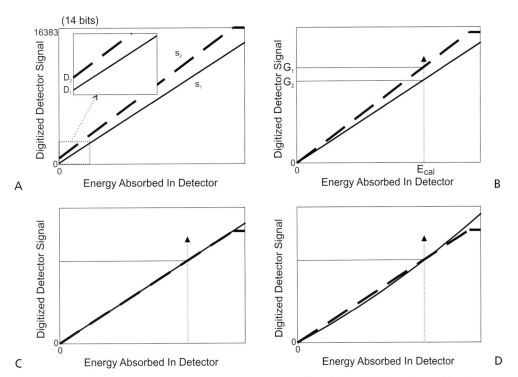

FIGURE 3-2. Correction for detector response nonuniformities. **(A)** A system with linear response illustrating two dels with different dark signals (intercepts) and gains (slopes). Enlarged view near the bottom end of the range, illustrates dark signals, D_1 and D_2. These are measured by acquiring images without radiation. **(B)** Response has been corrected for different dark signals. Gain is still different. Exposure to a fixed amount of radiation, E_{cal} allows determination of the slopes, G_1/E_{cal} and G_2/E_{cal} for each del. **(C)** Response of the dels after correction. **(D)** Systems with nonlinear response cannot be completely corrected using this simple method.

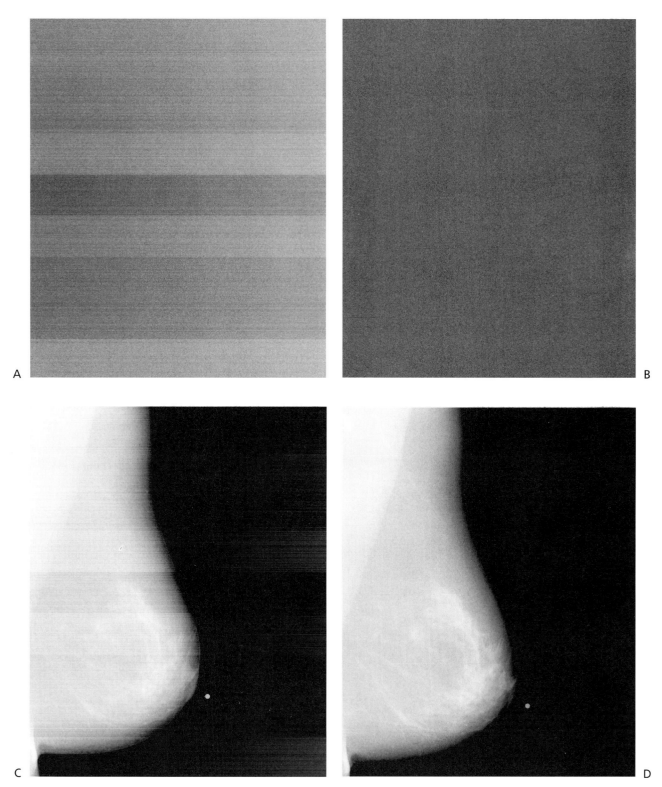

FIGURE 3-3. Example of the effect of flat-field correction. **(A)** Uncorrected image of a uniform attenuator. **(B)** Result after flat-field correction. **(C)** Uncorrected mammogram. **(D)** Mammogram with flat-fielding correction.

vidual mammogram. This can be most easily accomplished by averaging many acquired mask images together to form the working mask. For example, if the equivalent radiation for 10 images were used to form the mask, the noise in the mask would be reduced by $\sqrt{10}$, or about 3-fold, and the increase in noise because of flat-fielding would be 1.1 that of the uncorrected image (i.e., virtually unchanged).

Another point to remember is that the flat-fielding operation attempts to remove all spatial variation in what is assumed to be a uniform imaging field. But x-ray systems have many inherent nonuniformities in addition to those caused by the detector. These include the heel effect of the x-ray tube and the different path lengths that x-rays travel through air (inverse square law) and through the filter, compression plate, and grid, whose attenuation depends on the path length. Flat fielding will, therefore, remove the nonuniformity as a result of these other factors. It must be kept in mind that if imaging is performed with any of these factors altered (e.g., imaging at an energy other than where the flat fielding was performed or with a compression plate of a different thickness), the flat-fielding procedure may generate artifacts.

Although it is usually assumed that the detector has linear response to radiation, if there are minor nonlinearities and these are different from del to del, the detector may provide a highly uniform response when operated at the signal level at which flat fielding was performed. However, there may be nonuniformities when other intensities are employed. This will result in imperfect matching of response between dels at some intensities (Fig. 3-2d).

LINEAR VERSUS LOGARITHMIC RESPONSE

The transmission of x-rays along a particular path through the breast is given by:

$$n = n_0 e^{-\sum_{path} \mu(z)\Delta z}$$

where n is the number of x-rays transmitted and n_o the number incident, $\mu(z)$ is the attenuation coefficient for a tissue element of size Δz at location z. To simplify this expression, it has been assumed that the x-rays are monoenergetic. A detector having linear response produces a signal proportional to the number of x-rays transmitted and, therefore, exponentially related to the actual tissue properties. From an anatomical point of view, it may be desirable to measure not n, but its logarithm, so that the signal would be:

$$\log(n_0/n) = \sum_{path} \mu(z)\Delta z$$

which is more directly related to the tissue composition along the path.

This can be done by using a logarithmic amplifier to transform the signal from the detector. It provides the advantage of reducing the range of signal that must be digitized. However, it does make the flat-fielding offset and gain corrections substantially more difficult, as simple linear corrections can no longer be used.

DETECTOR TYPES

Currently there are several types of detectors used for digital mammography. They are briefly described here in Table 3-2.

Phosphor Flat Panel

This system (Fig. 3-4) consists of a large-area plate composed of amorphous silicon. Onto this plate a rectangular array of light-sensitive photodiodes is formed. X-rays are absorbed by a layer of thallium-activated cesium iodide phosphor CsI (Tl) deposited onto the photodiodes. The photodiodes, which constitute the dels of the detector, detect the light emitted by the phosphor and create an electrical charge signal that is stored on each del.

Because of its crystal structure, CsI has an advantage over the type of conventional phosphors used in screen-film imaging. This is illustrated in Figure 3-5. In a conventional phosphor (Figure 3-5A), the light quanta produced upon x-ray absorption readily move laterally, leading to increased width of the line-spread function. The CsI crystals (Figure 3-5B) can be grown to form needle-like or columnar structures that act as "light pipes" to reduce lateral spread. This allows the detector to be made thicker without as much resolution loss as would occur in those conventional phosphors.

TABLE 3-2. CURRENT DIGITAL MAMMOGRAPHY SYSTEMS

Model	Del size	Matrix size	Bit depth	Technology	Grid
Fischer Senoscan	50 µ	4 × 5.6K	12	CsI, CCDs, slot-scan	
Fuji CR	50 µ	4.7 × 6K	10 (log)	dual side CR	
GE 2000D	100 µ	2 × 2.3K	14	CsI on a-Si	
Lorad Selenia	70 µ	3 × 4K	14	a-Se	

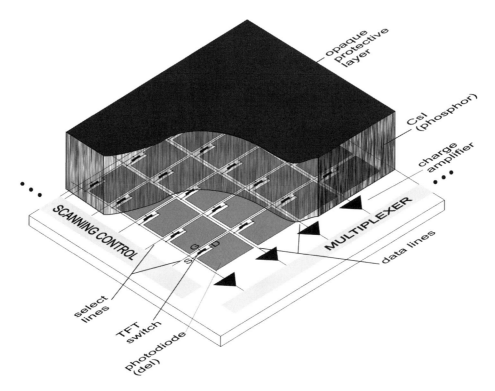

FIGURE 3-4. Concept of the CsI-amorphous silicon photodiode flat panel detector.

Each del on the array contains a photodiode and a thin film transistor (TFT) switch. There is a control line for each row of the array. These are sequentially energized to activate all the switches in that row. Along each column is a readout line, so that when a particular row is activated, the readout lines provide signal from all of the dels on that row.

In the system of this type, produced by General Electric Medical Systems (Milwaukee, WI) (Fig. 3-6), the del pitch is 100 μm, the field size is 19 cm × 23 cm and the digitization is carried out at 14 bits.

Uniformity correction with such detectors requires that a separate offset and sensitivity correction measurement is

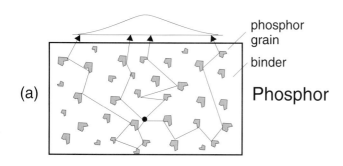

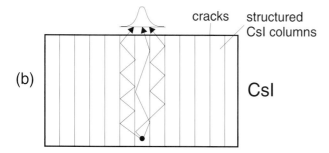

FIGURE 3-5. Advantage of CsI crystals for maintaining good spatial resolution while achieving high η. **(a)** In a conventional phosphor screen, light diverges strongly from its point of creation at the site of x-ray interaction. This gives rise to a broader point or line-spread function (shown above the phosphor screen). **(b)** With CsI, the light is channeled down the needlelike or columnar crystal formations, yielding a narrower PSF or LSF (i.e., a sharper image).

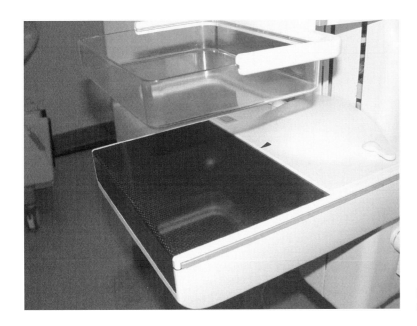

FIGURE 3-6. Photo of the detector housing of the GE digital mammography system.

stored for each del in the detector. Therefore, the number of such constants is equal to twice the number of dels in the detector. It is typical to remeasure offset values between images; however, the sensitivity matrix generally need only be measured occasionally.

Phosphor CCD System

This detector also uses a CsI(Tl) phosphor; however, in this case, it is deposited on a coupling plate consisting of millions of optical fibers. The fiber optics serve two roles. They conduct light from the phosphor to a charge-coupled device (CCD) array, which converts the light into an electronic signal that is digitized. In addition, the optical fibers stop much of the radiation that is not absorbed by the phosphor and thereby protect the CCD from the radiation damage that would result from direct exposure to x-rays. The fibers are arranged in an orderly array such that the pattern of light produced by the phosphor is conducted to the CCD with minimal spread.

The CCD is an electronic chip containing rows and columns of light-sensitive elements. These are arranged such that charge produced on each element in response to light exposure can be transferred down the columns of the CCD and read out on a single line. Generally 4 or 5 CCD chips are required to span the length of the detector.

In the current commercial implementation of this type of detector, the detector is a long, narrow rectangular shape, approximately 1 cm × 24 cm. The x-ray beam is collimated into a narrow slot to match this format (Fig. 3-7). To acquire the image, the x-ray beam and detector are scanned in synchrony across the breast. Charge created in the CCD is transferred down the columns from row to row at the same rate, but in an opposite direction to the physical motion of the

detector across the breast so that bundles of charge are integrated, collected, and read out corresponding to the x-ray transmission incident on the detector for each x-ray path through the breast. This is referred to as time-delay integration (TDI).

There are both advantages and disadvantages to the scanning approach. It requires a longer total image acquisition time than the area detector described above, and because most of the x-rays emitted by the tube are removed by the slot beam collimation, the x-ray tube heat loading is greater. On the other hand, there is an intrinsic high efficiency of scatter rejection so that a grid is not required and a dose reduction should be possible. Although there must be a specially designed scanning mechanism, the detector has fewer elements and should therefore be less expensive than a full-area detector.

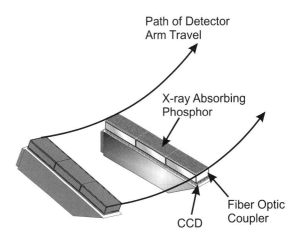

FIGURE 3-7. Schematic of detector used in a scanned slot TDI system.

Because all of the dels in a column of the detector participate in each image point measurement for that column the correction for offset and sensitivity need only be made for each column of the detector rather than for each del.

A scanning system of this type is marketed by Fischer Medical Imaging Corporation (Denver, CO). It employs dels of 54 μm. Over a limited portion of the detector, data can be read out at 27 μm intervals to provide a high-resolution mode. Digitization is performed at 12 bits.

Computed Radiography (CR) System

CR systems are widely used outside of mammography and employ a phosphor screen possessing a property called photostimulable luminescence as the x-ray absorber. Energy from x-ray absorption causes electrons in the phosphor crystal to be temporarily freed from the crystal matrix and then captured and stored in "traps" within the crystal lattice. The number of filled traps is proportional to the absorbed x-ray signal.

The image is then read out by placing the screen in a reader and scanning it with a red laser beam. This causes the electrons to be "knocked out" of the traps and to return to their original resting state. In doing so they may pass between energy levels in the crystal structure created by doping the crystal with certain materials. The difference in these energy levels corresponds to the energy of blue light, which is given off by the phosphor when such transitions occur. Thus the amount of blue light emitted and measured by an optical collecting system and a photomultiplier tube (Fig. 3-8A) is proportional to the energy of x-rays absorbed by the phosphor. A filter in the optical chain prevents the stimulating red light from interfering with the measurement.

There are no discrete dels on the phosphor plate itself. Rather, the time at which the laser beam strikes a given location on the screen gives the x–y coordinates of each

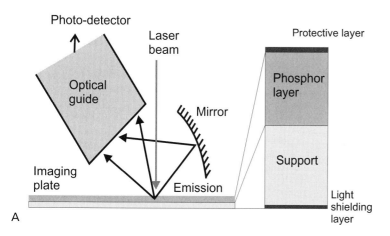

A

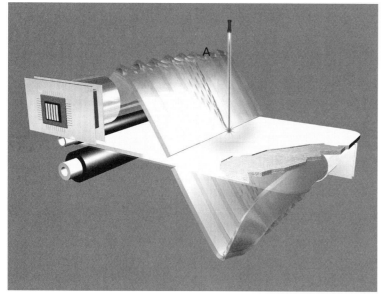

B

FIGURE 3-8. Photostimulable phosphor system. **(A)** Single side reader. **(B)** Double-sided reader. (Courtesy Fujifilm Medical Systems.)

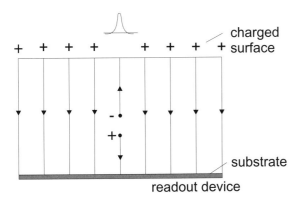

FIGURE 3-9. Schematic of a direct conversion photoconductive detector.

image location. In this system the spatial sampling is determined by the size of the laser spot (del size) and the distance between sample measurements (pitch).

A system of this type has been developed by Fujifilm Medical Systems (subsidiary of Fuji Photo Film Company, Ltd, Tokyo). In its original form, dels were of a nominal size of 100 μm. In such a system the spatial resolution is not degraded by spreading of the light emitted from the phosphor, because it is the size of the stimulating laser beam that determines the del size. On the other hand, scattering of the laser light in penetrating the phosphor screen to discharge the traps does cause blur because traps laterally displaced from the original path of the light also become discharged.

In addition, because collection of the light signal affects sensitivity, it is important that the light produced from the phosphor be collected efficiently. If an inadequate amount of light is measured from each interacting x-ray, then the image will contain additional noise above and beyond the quantum noise, causing the SNR and DQE to be reduced.

To improve the system, the manufacturer has refined the plate technology to reduce laser scattering, reduced the size of the laser spot to provide a nominal del size of 50 μm and increased the efficiency of light collection by reading from both the top and bottom surfaces of the phosphor plate (Fig. 3-8b).

Unlike the other systems, this system employs removable cassettes which can be used in the bucky tray of a standard mammography unit. While providing flexibility and economic advantages, this does necessitate that the plates be manually transported to the reader for processing. Although, by employing careful registration of each plate in the reader it should be possible to produce a sensitivity correction for each plate, this is currently not done. Therefore, with the current approach, the effects of "structure noise" on the plate are not removed. On the other hand, because these corrections are not performed, it is feasible for logarithmic digitization to be performed on this system.

Selenium Flat Panel

Unlike the previously described systems, this detector does not employ a phosphor; but instead, the x-ray absorber is composed of amorphous selenium. When this material absorbs x-rays, electric charge is liberated in the material in the form of electron-hole pairs. If electrodes are placed on the upper and lower surfaces of the selenium as in Figure 3-9 and an electric field is applied between the electrodes, then the charge signal can be collected onto a readout surface. This surface can be created on a plate of amorphous silicon in a manner similar to that of the phosphor flat plate system (Fig. 3-4). In this case, however, the photodiodes are replaced by a set of simple electrode pads to collect the charge, which is read out using TFT switches. A selenium system is currently produced by Lorad (Danbury, CT). Dels are 70 μm, with 14-bit digitization. A system is also being developed by Anrad (St Laurent, Quebec, Canada) with 85 μm dels (Fig. 3-10).

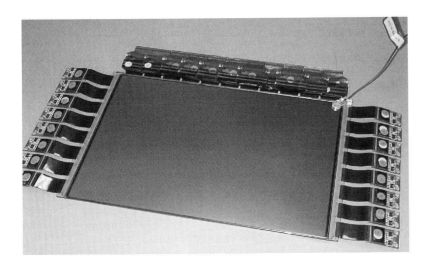

FIGURE 3-10. Amorphous selenium detector on amorphous silicon photodiode readout for digital mammography. (Photograph courtesy Anrad Corporation of St. Laurent, Quebec, Canada.)

X-Ray Quantum Counting Systems

All of the preceding systems operate on the principle of accumulating the signal from all of the x-rays that fall on a del during a particular exposure and digitizing this to form an element of the image. It is also possible to build x-ray detectors in which each interacting x-ray quantum is counted individually.

This approach has a few advantages. Previously, the effect on noise because of the variation in signal produced by an interacting x-ray was discussed. If, instead, the detector simply registers a count whenever an x-ray interacts, then no noise is associated with energy conversion, only the primary fluctuation of the number of quanta interacting with the detector. In addition, an x-ray produces exactly one count regardless of its energy. Some authors have argued that the standard x-ray detector places a higher weight on the higher energy x-rays that interact, because these produce more light, but less contrast. Quantum counting removes this weighting.

The greatest challenge for quantum counting systems is to be able to accommodate the high rate of x-rays interacting per second in each del. For the unattenuated beam, this can be 10^6 quanta/s or higher. Modern electronics can now handle these rates. In the future, it may also be feasible to take this approach another step forward and analyze the energy carried by each interacting quantum and weight the signals thus produced to provide optimum information.

Currently two quantum counting systems are under development. Both are based on the principle of a linear detector; however, to acquire an image in a reasonably short time, both systems use multiple line detectors and move them during acquisition to fully cover the image plane. This necessitates extremely precise motion control to avoid gaps or overlap when stitching the image together.

The first system, by Sectra (Stockholm) employs crystalline silicon crystals as direct x-ray absorbers (Fig. 3-11). The charge produced from each interacting x-ray is collected in an electric field and shaped into a pulse, which is counted. In the second system, built by XCounter (Stockholm), the x-rays interact with a high pressure gas inside the detector vessel and the ions produced are used to form the pulse (Fig. 3-12).

SPATIAL RESOLUTION

The spatial resolution characteristics of each detector type are somewhat different. In the CsI(Tl) systems, light produced in the phosphor attempts to spread isotropically from the point of emission. The CsI crystals tend to channel the light down the length of the crystal by total internal reflection and to some extent this mitigates the spread of light. Nevertheless, as the detector is made thicker to increase η, there is more spreading of light and a decrease in spatial resolution.

In the CR system, the spatial localization is determined by the laser and, therefore, the spread of light emitted from the phosphor is not important. On the other hand, the laser light that scans the plate scatters on entering the phosphor material causing traps laterally displaced from the point of incidence to be discharged and to contribute to the signal. This can have a marked effect in reducing resolution and

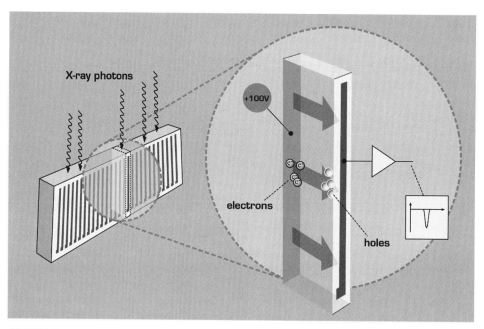

FIGURE 3-11. X-ray counting detector based on silicon. (Photograph courtesy Sectra, Stockholm.)

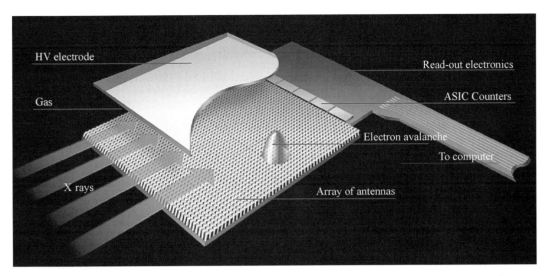

FIGURE 3-12. High pressure gaseous x-ray counting detector. (Photo courtesy Xcounter, Stockholm.)

the effect becomes increasingly important as the thickness of the plate increases. Therefore, with these systems there is a trade-off between η and spatial resolution.

This issue becomes much less important in the direct conversion detector. The charge signal is moved quickly toward the collection electrode by the electric field before the charge has much opportunity to spread. Therefore, by appropriate choice of electric field, the resolution can be maintained at a high level while at the same time keeping the detector thickness large enough to ensure high resolution. Sample MTFs of these systems are presented in Figure 3-13. Because factors other than the del aperture, d, affect the MTF, the ordering of the curves does not necessarily correlate with the del sizes.

AUTOMATIC EXPOSURE CONTROL

Digital image acquisition provides enormous opportunities for automatic optimization of image acquisition. For example, it is no longer necessary to have a separate AEC sensor as part of the system because the digital detector can serve as a multielement sensor. To use the detector in this way, it is necessary that the detector can be read out quickly to determine what the optimum exposure factors should be. This may impose difficulty for some of the current detectors and creative ways of accomplishing this will have to be found.

Optimization of exposure can consider various statistics from a short test pulse made prior to the actual image

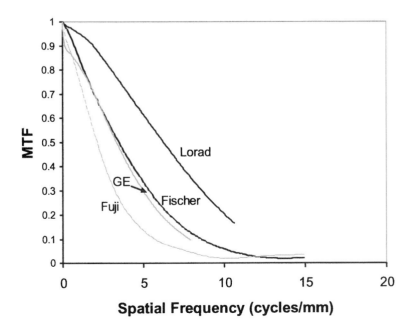

FIGURE 3-13. MTFs of some current digital mammography systems.

acquisition. These might include the minimum signal from the most attenuating region of the breast. The algorithm can require that in the actual exposure, this signal be greater than some preset value. Alternatively, the SDNR can be predicted, and the exposure can be planned to achieve no less than a certain SDNR in any part of the image. Additional data on the compression thickness and force can also be used to refine the algorithm. These opportunities are only beginning to be realized today and exploiting them remains an exciting challenge for researchers and system designers.

SUGGESTED READINGS

1. Swank RK. Absorption and noise in x-ray phosphors. J Appl Phys 1973;44:4199–4203.
2. Yaffe MJ, Rowlands JA. X-ray detectors for digital radiography. Phys Med Biol 1997;42:1–39.

4

DIGITAL MAMMOGRAPHY CLINICAL TRIALS

ETTA D. PISANO

HISTORY OF FOOD AND DRUG ADMINISTRATION APPROVAL OF DIGITAL MAMMOGRAPHY

On June 19, 1996, the FDA published *Information for Manufacturers Seeking Marketing Clearance of Digital Mammography Systems*. It outlined a requirement that manufacturers conduct a clinical trial designed to show agreement between screen-film mammography and digital mammography if devices were to become FDA-approved through the 510(k) or Premarket Approval (PMA) mechanism. Manufacturers were instructed to discuss the proposed investigational plans with the FDA's Center for Devices and Radiological Health (CDRH).

The FDA specifically indicated within its guidance document that the probability of a positive digital mammogram should be greater than 0.90 if the screen-film mammogram were positive and the probability of a negative digital mammogram should be greater than 0.95 if the screen-film mammogram were negative. In addition, the FDA estimated that 520 women (260 with abnormal screen-film mammograms and 260 with normal screen-film mammograms) would be needed in a trial to achieve such an estimate of agreement. There was no requirement that manufacturers determine truth about the presence or absence of cancer in the patient, only that the screen-film mammogram interpretations and the digital mammogram interpretations agree.

All digital mammography manufacturers designed agreement studies, which were discussed extensively with the CDRH. Recruitment to clinical trials was begun shortly thereafter. The trials that were carried out were quite similar, as would be expected, because the FDA provided a blueprint for the manufacturers to follow.

Unfortunately, the FDA's guidelines were flawed in that the level of agreement required for digital mammography with screen-film mammography was not attainable, even when screen-film mammography was compared to itself, because of intra- and interreader variability (1–3).

This issue was discussed at a meeting of the Advisory Panel convened by the FDA on August 17, 1998. On February 8, 1999, the FDA revised its guidance document and notified the manufacturers that the clinical section was no longer valid. Letters were sent to all of the manufacturers indicating that the digital mammography FDA approval trials would now be required to be based on truth regarding breast cancer status and not direct agreement with screen-film mammography. That is to say, sensitivity and specificity, as measured by a methodology like Receiver Operating Characteristic (ROC) analysis, were intrinsic to the trials and had to be included in reports to the FDA for approval purposes.

All manufacturers subsequently negotiated with the FDA on protocol revisions so as to meet these new requirements. Their subsequent efforts centered on conducting reader studies using sets of mammograms that contain multiple cases with biopsy-proven lesions. This involved enrolling additional women or collecting additional cases from the existent databases at participating centers. The goal of these studies was to show that the difference in area under the ROC curve between digital and film was no greater than 0.1. This was the FDA's standard for proving "substantial equivalence" of the two technologies.

General Electric (GE) presented data to an FDA panel on December 16, 1999. Postmarket approval (PMA) of the GE unit was granted on January 31, 2000. GE subsequently received FDA approval for its softcopy display system for digital mammography in November 2000. Similarly, Fischer received FDA approval for both hard and softcopy versions of its imaging system in late September 2001, and Lorad's CCD-based system received approval for hardcopy display in the Spring of 2002. In October 2002, Hologic, Inc. (Bedford, MA), Lorad's parent company, received FDA approval for its selenium-based digital detector for both softcopy and printed film display, based on a claim of substantial equivalence with the Lorad product.

Other companies undergoing FDA trials for their digital mammography devices are Fujifilm Medical Systems (a subsidiary of Fuji Photo Film Company, Tokyo), Sectra (Stockholm), Instrumentarium (Tuusula, Finland), and Xcounter (Stockholm).

General Electric FDA Trial

Edward Hendrick of the University of Colorado led the GE Senographe 2000D FDA approval trial. In that study, 625 women aged 40 and over, presenting for diagnostic mammography at the University of Colorado, the University of Massachusetts, Massachusetts General Hospital, and the University of Pennsylvania, underwent both digital and screen-film mammography. Radiation doses were equalized between the two systems. Images were interpreted independently by five radiologists. The recall rate of digital mammography was statistically significantly lower than the recall rate of screen-film by 2% (p > 0.001) whether all cases or only noncancer cases were considered (i.e., 46.9% vs. 48.8% and 45.4% vs. 47.3%, respectively). Specificity was 55% for digital and 53% for screen-film. Sensitivity was 68% for digital and 70% for screen-film (p = 0.0245)(4).

Fischer Medical Imaging SenoScan FDA Trial

The Fischer SenoScan FDA Trial, led by Etta D. Pisano of the University of North Carolina (UNC), used screen-film and digital mammograms of 676 women, who were scheduled for biopsy at six centers (UNC, Brooke Army Hospital, Sally Jobe Breast Center (CO), Thomas Jefferson University, the University of California at San Francisco, and the University of Toronto). Eight radiologists read a subset of these mammograms: 111 of women with cancer and 136 with negative findings. The average area under the ROC curve for that study was 0.715 for digital and 0.765 for screen-film mammography. The sensitivity of screen-film and digital mammography were 0.74 and 0.66 respectively. The specificities were 0.60 for screen-film mammography and 0.67 for digital (5).

FEDERALLY FUNDED CLINICAL TRIALS ON DIGITAL MAMMOGRAPHY

Four large federally funded clinical trials have been opened as of August 1, 2002. Two of the trials compare digital mammography to screen-film mammography for the screening mammography population, one just for the GE system and the other for five different machine types. The other two trials will compare digital mammography to screen-film mammography for the diagnostic mammography population, utilizing reader studies at the end of enrollment to assess the relative diagnostic accuracy of the two modalities.

DIGITAL MAMMOGRAPHY SCREENING TRIALS

Department of Defense General Electric Screening Trial

The only federally funded clinical screening trial that has been completed and published to date was funded by the Department of Defense (Edward Hendrick, University of Colorado (UC), PI) and utilized only GE digital mammography equipment. This study enrolled 4,945 women over age 40 presenting for screening mammography at two centers, UC and the University of Massachusetts (Carl D'Orsi, University of Massachusetts Medical Center (UMMC), co-PI). The unique aspect of this study is that the workup of lesions proceeded based on the findings of either digital or screen-film mammography. This is a significant strength of this study, as it allows for cancers to be detected by either modality (6).

In this trial, over a 30-month enrollment period, 6,736 paired screen-film and digital mammography examinations were performed on 4,489 women. There were 179 biopsies leading to the diagnosis of 50 cancers, 42 detected through imaging and 8 interval malignancies. This study revealed that there was no statistically significant difference in sensitivity or area under the ROC curve for the two modalities.

Table 4-1 shows the breakdown of cancer detection by modality for this trial (6). There were more cancers missed by digital mammography than by film (23 for digital vs. 17 for film, out of 50 cancers total). The sensitivities for digital and screen-film mammography in this study were 54% and 66% respectively. The area under the ROC curve was 0.74 for digital mammography and 0.80 for screen-film mammography. Again, neither of these small differences was significant.

The lead radiologists for this study believe that the difference in small number of cancers that were visible with digital that were not visible by film (and vice versa) were *not* the result of the differences between the modalities per se, but were the result of small differences in compression and positioning that could not be held constant across the performance of the two studies, despite the fact that the examinations were usually performed by the same technologist within a very short time interval (7).

TABLE 4-1. CANCERS DETECTED IN DOD SCREENING TRIAL (6)

Modality		Screen-film mammography	
		Yes	No
	Was the cancer found?		
Digital mammography	Yes	18	9
	No	15	8

In addition, this study also showed that digital mammography had a statistically significantly lower recall rate (11.8% vs. 14.9%, p<0.001), and a statistically significantly lower number of biopsies recommended than were recommended because of abnormal screen-film mammography (94 for digital mammography vs. 143 for screen-film mammography).

In this trial, all digital cases were read using softcopy display. It is possible that the reduced false–positive rate for digital compared to screen-film mammography was because of this factor. That is to say, immediate manipulation of the image allowed for some on-line assessment of areas of concern that would ordinarily have required another patient visit and additional mammographic views. It is also possible, however, that the nonsignificant trend toward reduced sensitivity of the GE system is the result of reduced spatial resolution in general of digital versus film. This would allow for the detection of fewer findings, both benign and malignant, that would have the effect of improved specificity, as most mammographic findings are benign.

The Digital Mammographic Imaging Screening Trial (DMIST)

The American College of Radiology Imaging Network (ACRIN), funded by the National Cancer Institute (NCI) in March 1999, is a cooperative group formed to perform multiinstitutional clinical trials of diagnostic imaging and imaging-guided therapeutic technologies. Similar to the other clinical trials organizations supported by the NCI, this organization will develop and support interdisciplinary research on the use of imaging technology in the diagnosis and treatment of cancer. ACRIN trials will evaluate both traditional radiological outcome measures, such as sensitivity, specificity, and area under the receiver operating characteristic (ROC) curve, and less traditional metrics, such as cost effectiveness and other patient-centered outcomes, such as quality of life and satisfaction. NCI originally awarded ACRIN over $22 million for a five-year period, 1999 through 2004.

Bruce Hillman, MD, of the University of Virginia, serves as the Principal Investigator for ACRIN. He is responsible for developing and leading the committees that promote the scientific activities of the network. The ACR research office in Philadelphia, headed by Thomas Caldwell, MBA, MHSA, serves as the headquarters for ACRIN. That facility serves as the data and image storage repository for all ACRIN trials. In addition, as it has for the Radiation Therapy Oncology Group (RTOG) for its first 25 years, ACR staff supports protocol development and handles quality assurance, auditing, informatics, logistics, and financial management. Constantine Gatsonis, PhD, of Brown University, heads the biostatistical and data management center for ACRIN. He and his colleagues oversee protocol design and data analysis, as well as supervise data management activities at ACRIN headquarters in Philadelphia (8).

In October 2001, ACRIN opened DMIST, which is funded by the NCI. This trial includes five available digital mammography machine types to allow for a generic statement about the diagnostic accuracy of digital mammography versus screen-film mammography in a screening population.

The primary aim of the study is to evaluate the diagnostic accuracy of digital mammography versus screen-film mammography in the population of patients presenting for screening mammography. All participants undergo both digital and screen-film mammography. Each study will be independently interpreted. Workup of abnormalities will proceed based on the findings of both examinations. In this manner, the digital and screen-film mammograms may both lead to the detection of unsuspected cancers. The breast cancer status of all participants will be determined by histological evaluation of all lesions recommended for biopsy, and by clinical follow-up, including mammography one year after entry into the study (9).

The study includes five of the major digital mammography machines available for clinical testing or purchase in the U.S. These are the General Electric Senographe 2000D (General Electric Medical Systems, Milwaukee), the Fischer Imaging SenoScan (Fischer Imaging Corporation, Denver), the Trex Digital Mammography System (Trex Medical Corporation, Stamford, CT), Fuji Computed Radiography (Fuji Medical Systems, Stamford, CT) and the Hologic amorphous selenium digital mammography system (Hologic, Inc., Bedford, MA). There are 35 U.S. and Canadian sites participating in this trial. The total accrual target for this trial is 49,500 women.

The cases that are accrued as part of this trial will serve as a valuable resource to future investigators. The image data will be available to other ACRIN investigators and industry to assist in the development of new Computer Aided Diagnosis/Detection (CAD) and image processing algorithms.

One of the strongest aspects of DMIST is all devices are expected to meet rigorous quality control standards. In this way, much as the MQSA sets standards for all different types of screen-film mammography systems, similar standards are being followed so that the machine differences can be reduced. This will allow statements regarding the benefits of digital mammography versus screen-film mammography when both technologies meet high quality control standards. More details about the QC procedures utilized in DMIST are provided in Chapter 5.

Two potential confounders for all clinical digital mammography trials are the display method (softcopy vs. printed film) and image processing algorithms applied to all images. Selecting the appropriate image processing for display of the digital mammograms is important and may significantly affect the outcome of all clinical trials involving digital mammography. Whatever is used should be standardized across all readers for each machine type within any trial. This is being accomplished within DMIST by working closely with the manufacturers to assure that all readers across all centers have access to any new image processing at the same time. In addition, the method of display, softcopy or printed film, is being controlled within each system. All Fuji and Trex images are being read on printed film as much as possible. GE readers read softcopy only. Fischer cases are read with *both* softcopy and printed film display. Hologic readers read either softcopy or printed film. In addition, there will be a large reader study at the end of the accrual period when the digital cases will be read in a controlled fashion for comparison of softcopy versus printed film display within each system.

The trial will also assess the relative cost effectiveness of digital and screen-film mammography and the effect on other patient outcomes, such as the quality of life as a result of the expected reduction in false positives with digital mammography. In addition, through a series of reader studies at the end of the trial, the cases accrued will be utilized to evaluate the effect of disease prevalence on reader interpretation performance, the effect of breast density on the diagnostic accuracy of digital mammography versus screen-film mammography, and, the diagnostic accuracy of each of the five individual digital mammography units versus screen-film mammography.

Finally, for prior breast cancer screening trials, mortality from breast cancer has served as the most important outcome measure. This is neither possible nor realistic for digital mammography. The window of opportunity for performing such a study is quite narrow. Now that digital mammography is FDA approved, it will gradually become widely available. The longer the delay in opening a screening trial, the higher would be the probability that the results would be confounded by crossover of patients between the two systems and noncompliance with randomization assignment. Surrogate endpoints, such as those selected in the DOD and ACRIN screening studies, that is, sensitivity and specificity, positive and negative predictive values, and ROC curve differences, are practical and realistic for future screening trials for digital mammography.

DIGITAL MAMMOGRAPHY TRIALS INCLUDING PATIENTS WITH PROBLEMS

Office of Women's Health Diagnostic Mammography Study

The first diagnostic mammography trial, funded by the Office of Women's Health, was run under the auspices of the International Digital Mammography Development Group (IDMDG) (Etta D. Pisano, UNC, PI) and enrolled 201 women at eight centers. Table 4-2 lists the centers involved in this study, the principal investigator at each site, and the type of digital mammography unit used at that site. Two patient cohorts were enrolled, Group A and Group B.

Group A consisted of all consecutive women with mammographically dense breasts who presented to the participating mammography clinics for problem-solving mammography and who were scheduled to undergo either open or percutaneous large-core needle breast biopsy within the 12 weeks after the eligibility mammogram. Women with palpable and/or nonpalpable lesions were included in this group.

Group B consisted of a random sample of women with mammographically dense breasts who presented to the participating mammography clinics for problem-solving mammography, who were not scheduled to undergo biopsy, and who were recommended for one-year follow-up.

Eighteen radiologist readers interpreted images, either in screen-film format, manufacturer's printed digital format (default) or in digital processed format with Histogram-based Intensity Windowing (HIW) or Contrast Limited Adaptive Histogram Equalization (CLAHE) image processing. Readers scored all cases using a six-point scale and ROC analysis was utilized. Baseline reader performance with screen-film were obtained through the additional interpretation of 179 UNC screen-film mammograms, matched by lesion type, breast density, and cancer status to digital cases. A repeated measures analysis of covariance allowing unequal slopes was used in each of nine analyses (AUC, sensitivity, and specificity for each of three machine types).

The reading of the film mammograms from the same patients was not performed in this study, but a comparable

TABLE 4-2. OFFICE OF WOMEN'S HEALTH CLINICAL TRIAL

Institution	Machine type	PI
University of Pennsylvania	GE	Emily Conant
Massachusetts General Hospital	GE	Daniel Kopans
University of Toronto	Fischer	Rene Shumak
Mount Sinai Hospital	Fischer	Roberta Jong
Thomas Jefferson	Trex	Stephen Feig
University of North Carolina	Fischer	Etta D. Pisano
Good Samaritan Hospital (NY)	Trex	Melinda Staiger
University of Virginia	Trex	Laurie Fajardo

set of screen-film mammogram was used to establish reader performance. This study showed that sensitivity, specificity and area under the ROC curve probably varies by lesion type and image processing algorithim selected, although the differences were not statistically significant (10). The comparison of film to digital mammography interpretation directly using the Office of Women's Health cases was subsequently undertaken under separate funding from the Komen Foundation. Those results are pending.

This study served as a pilot study for another larger clinical trial, funded by the Department of Defense (Laurie Fajardo, University of Iowa, PI), which opened for accrual in July 2000. An additional 1,075 women in essentially the same patient cohorts are being enrolled at seven centers. Table 4-3 shows the institutions and investigators involved and the type of digital mammography equipment that will be utilized at each site. A larger reader study of all 1,275 cases will take place at the end of accrual.

Both of these diagnostic mammography studies are somewhat limited by the fact that they rely on the presence of physical examination findings or an abnormal screen-film mammogram to select eligible patients. This may cause an underestimate of the diagnostic accuracy of digital mammography. An underestimate of the efficacy of digital mammography is possible because of the study design, because some patients enter the study by virtue of the visibility of their breast lesions on screen-film mammography but no patients enter the study by virtue of the visibility of their breast lesions on digital mammography. Therefore, it would be difficult for digital mammography to perform better than screen-film mammography in such a population.

Other Published Clinical Studies of Digital Mammography in the Diagnostic Setting

Hundertmark and his colleagues performed 100 digital screening mammograms and 50 spot magnification views and compared his findings with those from screen-film mammograms on the same patients. He concluded that the diagnostic value of digital mammograms using direct magnification technique is comparable to standard mammography with regard to the identification of calcifications. In

86% of the cases, calcifications were seen on both modalities. In 8% of the cases, additional calcifications were detected on digital that had not been seen on screen-film. Fourfold spot magnification views provided improved detection of calcifications, with the digital magnification technique providing an additional 26% detection rate over the conventional analog technique (11).

Grebe and colleagues compared more than 1,000 GE digital mammograms with conventional mammograms. These authors reported that DM provided better visualization of the skin and subcutaneous structures, as well as microcalcifications in very dense glandular tissue, in irradiated tissue after breast cancer surgery and in dense breasts of young women. These authors believed that the high-contrast resolution in the digital system and the use of appropriate softcopy intensity windowing improved the visualization of calcifications against dense backgrounds (12). Similar cases are given in Chapter 12.

Venta and colleagues have studied the rate and cause of disagreements in interpretation between GE digital and film mammograms in a diagnostic setting by asking radiologists to independently assign ACR BIRADS codes to more than 1,100 paired mammograms. Agreement between digital and film interpretations was achieved in 82%, partial agreement in 14%, and disagreement in 4%, for a kappa value of 0.29. Screening mammograms had a higher rate of agreement than diagnostic mammograms (87% vs. 70%) and a lower rate of disagreement (2% vs. 7%) than diagnostic mammograms (p<0.0001). The primary causes of disagreement between digital and screen-film interpretations of diagnostic mammograms were differences in management approach between radiologists (interobserver variability) (52%), information from additional FSM images or ultrasound images of suspicious lesions (34%), and technical differences in the examinations (10%) (13).

Hildell and colleagues compared Fuji CR mammography to screen-film mammography in terms of visibility and detectability of details of the breast parenchyma in a series of 1,200 women examined with both techniques. These authors reported that the appearance of irregular calcifications as well as smoothly rounded benign and "probably benign" calcifications was clearly appreciated with both modalities. They also noted that evaluation of dense breasts

TABLE 4-3. DEPARTMENT OF DEFENSE CENTER CLINICAL TRIAL

Institution	Machine type	PI
Johns Hopkins University	Trex/Hologic	Laurie Fajardo
University of Iowa	Trex/Hologic	Laurie Fajardo
University of Pennsylvania	GE	Emily Conant
University of Toronto	Fischer	Roberta Jong
University of North Carolina	Fischer and GE	Etta D. Pisano
Good Samaritan Hospital (NY)	Trex	Melinda Staiger
University of California, LA	GE	Lawrence Bassett

was often easier on digital images, and the skin and the subcutaneous tissue could be evaluated without using high-intensity illumination. Unfortunately, this study is limited by the lack of detail on its methodology (14).

SUMMARY

Although digital mammography holds great promise, it is important that radiologists insist on evidence that it produces results of equivalent diagnostic accuracy to screen-film mammography, both in the screening and diagnostic settings, before it supplants the traditional technology. Given the ongoing clinical trials that are already underway, such evidence is expected by early 2006, at the latest. Third-party payers are likely to require such proof before substantially increasing reimbursement for this promising new technology.

REFERENCES

1. Howard DH, Elmore JG, Lee CH, et al. Observer variability in mammography. Trans Assoc Am Physicians 1993;106:96–100.
2. Elmore JG, Wells CK, Lee CH, et al. Variability in radiologists' interpretations of mammograms. N Engl J Med 1994;331(22): 1493–1499.
3. Beam CA, Layde PM, Sullivan DC. Variability in the interpretation of screening mammograms by US radiologists. Findings from a national sample. Arch Intern Med 1996;156(2):209–213.
4. Hendrick RE, Lewin JM, D'Orsi CJ, et al. Non-inferiority study of FFDM in an enriched diagnostic cohort: Comparison with screen-film mammography in 625 women. In: Yaffe MJ, ed. IWDM 2000: 5th International Workshop on Digital Mammography. Madison, WI: Medical Physics Publishing:2001; 475–481.
5. Cole EB, Pisano ED, Hanna LG, et al. Multicenter Clinical Assessment of the Fischer SenoScan Digital Mammography System. (abstract). Radiology (supplement) 2001;221(P):285.
6. Lewin JM, D'Orsi CJ, Hendrick RE, et al. Clinical Comparison of Full Field Digital Mammography and Screen-film Mammography for detection of breast cancer. AJR 1002;179: 671–677.
7. Lewin JM, Hendrick RE, D'Orsi CJ, et al. Comparison of full-field digital mammography with screen-film mammography for cancer detection: Results of 4,945 paired examinations. Radiology 2001;218:873–880.
8. Hillman BJ, Gatsonis C, Sullivan DC. American College of Radiology Imaging Network: New National Cooperative Group for Conducting Clinical Trials of Medical Imaging Technologies. Radiology 1999;213:641–645.
9. Galen B, Staab E, Pisano ED. The American College of Radiology Imaging Network: Digital Mammographic Imaging Screening Trial (DMIST): An update. Acad Radiol 2002;9:374–375.
10. Cole EB, Pisano ED, Kistner EO, et al. Diagnostic accuracy of digital mammography in patients with dense breasts presenting for problem-solving mammogaphy-Image processing and lesion type effects. Radiology 2003;226:153–160.
11. Hundertmark C, Breiter N, Hermann KP, et al. Digitale VergröBerungsmammographie in Speicherfolientechnik. Erste klinische Ergebnisse. Radiologe 1997;37(8):597–603.
12. Grebe S, Diekmann F, Bick U, et al. Erste klinische Erfahrungen mit der digitalen Vollfeldmammographie. Zentralbl Gynakol 2000;122(11):589–594.
13. Venta LA, Hendrick RE, Adler YT, et al. Rates and causes of disagreement in interpretation of full-field digital mammography and film-screen mammography in a diagnostic setting. Am J Roentgenol 2001;176(5):1241–1248.
14. Hildell J, Hofer B, Zynamon A. Storage phosphor digital mammography vs. screen-film mammography. Preliminary results of comparison in a phantom model and initial clinical experience. Radiol Diagn 1992;33(5):312–319.

5

QUALITY CONTROL FOR DIGITAL MAMMOGRAPHY

MARTIN J. YAFFE

QUALITY CONTROL FOR DIGITAL MAMMOGRAPHY

Mammography equipment is carefully designed to provide the best possible image quality at acceptable radiation doses. To realize this high performance, the equipment must be properly set up on installation and be maintained at this level throughout its use. This is accomplished through initial acceptance testing and a program of periodic quality control tests.

Because of the high public profile of breast cancer and of mammography as the best established means for its preclinical detection, in 1992 federal legislation mandated quality control (QC) for screen-film mammography in the United States under the Mammography Quality Standards Act (MQSA). Mammography is unique in being the only radiological examination to be regulated in this way. Prior to this, a voluntary program for accreditation of mammography facilities had been operated by the American College of Radiology (ACR). This program included a requirement for quality control testing, with specific test procedures carried out at specified regular intervals and with duties to be performed by the mammographic technologist, the radiologist, and the medical physicist. Under MQSA, accreditation by the ACR or one of four other FDA approved state accreditation bodies in the United States is mandatory. Accreditation requires performance of the QC program at an acceptable level. In most cases, MQSA performance standards are the same as those required by the ACR program at the time the legislation came into force. The ACR program was extremely beneficial because some facilities were performing studies that were of inadequate quality to permit detecting and/or diagnosing cancer. Prior to accreditation, there was no way a woman could have confidence that the quality of her mammographic examination was adequate.

The QC tests include the following:

1. Evaluation of the overall mechanical and electrical integrity of the mammography system.
2. Assessment of x-ray collimation and alignment of system.
3. Assessment of focal spot resolution.
4. Accuracy of kV.
5. Beam quality.
6. Performance of the automatic exposure control.
7. Uniformity of the sensitivity of the screens.
8. Radiation dose.
9. Viewing conditions.
10. Image quality and artifacts.

Performance of the QC tests monitors changes in the function of these components. Action levels are specified at which point adjustment, repair, or replacement of components is required to re-establish proper operation.

Quality control is essential for maintaining the imaging performance of a mammography system. However, QC involves costs because of the human labor required to perform the tests and the downtime of the mammography equipment during testing. Therefore, a well-designed QC program will incorporate tests that are relevant in that they are predictive of future degradation of imaging performance. These tests will also be done at a frequency that is high enough to intercept most drifts in quality or performance before they become diagnostically significant, but at the same time is reasonable with respect to the expected mean time between failures of these functions and the cost of QC. Some of the tests currently performed are not very useful in predicting failure, because modern generators tend to fail catastrophically, rather than because of gradual drifts.

DIGITAL MAMMOGRAPHY

At the time of this writing, the first accreditation program for digital mammography is being implemented by the ACR. Currently four types of digital mammography systems have received approval from the Food and Drug Administration (FDA) for clinical use in the United States. Although these do not comply with the accreditation program in place for screen-film systems, FDA allows them to be operated under a temporary exemption from the regulations. For example, to operate a digital mammography system, a facility must already have an accredited screen-film system in operation. In addition, the required QC program is substantially that provided by the manufacturer of each digital mammography system, as well as those of the manufacturers of applicable subsystems, such as softcopy displays and laser printers. Therefore, the type of QC that must be done in a facility that has two or more different types of digital mammography systems will vary with each system. Manufacturers' initial QC programs were designed to emulate most of the tests developed for screen-film mammography, with similar frequencies for performance of the tests. In many cases, manufacturers have not yet had adequate time and field experience with their equipment to determine the expected mean time between failures. This information is critical in establishing appropriate testing frequencies in a QC program. At present, no uniformity of test procedures exists among manufacturers.

Because each of the current digital mammography systems is different in design, the ACR has been required to introduce specialized accreditation programs for each system. These are being introduced one at a time in the order that the systems were approved by the FDA. While it is realized that there are fundamental differences in how different systems operate and that this will no doubt imply variations in the test procedures, it is desirable to create a set of procedures that is as generic across the spectrum of equipment as possible.

While digital mammography is not a radically different modality from its predecessor, there is good reason to believe that the approach to QC control should differ in some aspects. In screen-film mammography, the processed image must attain a certain target optical density to produce optimal display contrast. If this is not the case, the image quality will deteriorate markedly because of high local gradient at the optimum optical density and steep falloff in gradient at lower and higher optical densities (ODs) (see Fig. 2-4). For this reason, considerable effort is devoted in the QC process to the factors responsible for film OD, such as the sensitivity of the screens, the film processing parameters, and the automatic exposure control. In addition, because the imaging system does not produce quantitative information, tests of these functions must be done using external measuring equipment.

Digital mammography offers some clear advantages in its performance as compared to screen-film mammography. Because display brightness and contrast can be adjusted completely independently from image acquisition, the signal level produced by the system from an exposure is not particularly important in terms of how the image will appear. The exposure *does* affect the noise level of the digi-

tal image. Therefore, it is important that all relevant anatomy is imaged within the dynamic range of the recording system and that the signal-to-noise ratio (SNR) in the image is adequate for all parts of the breast.

ELEMENTS OF A DIGITAL MAMMOGRAPHY SYSTEM

The physics of digital mammography was reviewed in Chapter 2. However, it is probably useful to consider the system in terms of functional modules listed here.

1. The x-ray generator.
2. The x-ray tube and beam filtration.
3. The x-ray collimation.
4. The compression device.
5. The antiscatter grid (if applicable).
6. The detector, digitization, and automatic exposure control.
7. The acquisition workstation.
8. Interconnection to Picture Archiving and Communication System (PACS).
9. The review workstation.
10. The hard copy device.

Each of these components has a role in affecting the quality of the image and must perform in an optimal, predictable, and consistent manner. Although some components are extremely stable once set up, others may have a tendency to drift gradually in performance.

QUALITY CONTROL IN THE DIGITAL MAMMOGRAPHY IMAGE SCREENING TRIAL

For the Digital Mammography Imaging Screening Trial (DMIST), discussed in Chapter 4, an extensive QC program was especially developed to ensure a reasonable standard of performance of the digital systems at the 32 screening sites. During the course of the trial, five different types of digital mammography systems were employed. The QC program included a set of tests, test objects and phantoms, and a QC manual. The tests accommodated differences in the manner in which these systems operated. In addition, although they were developed independently from the programs of any of the manufacturers, the tests were designed to minimize repetition of testing, because to conform with MQSA, the facilities also had to carry out all of the tests described in the manufacturer's manual.

A radiograph of the phantom, "MISTY," is shown in Figure 5-1. At the time the study began, there was little experience with digital mammography. As a result, the

FIGURE 5-1. The MISTY phantom used in the DMIST trial.

phantom was designed to incorporate a wide variety of tests, knowing that some would probably later be found to be impractical, redundant, or not providing useful information. As part of the QC program, the Mammographic Accreditation Phantom, introduced for screen-film mammography by the ACR and illustrated schematically in Figure 5-2 was imaged on a daily basis. It was found that this phantom was not very helpful in distinguishing among different levels of image quality. In more than 4,000 total phantom images from the first 19 facilities in the trial, there were only four failures using the standards established for screen-film mammography. When we considered the possibility of increasing the requirements to specify how many fibers, speck groups, or masses had to be detectible (again by ACR evaluation methods), the failure rate immediately increased. For example, screen-film mammography must be able to visualize 4 fibers, 3 speck groups, and 3 masses. When this was changed to 4, 3.5, and 3, the failure rate increased to more than 20%! The gradation in size and the SNR provided by the structures was not sufficiently subtle to provide a scale on which to assess image quality. In general, existing subjective image-quality phantoms designed for screen-film mammography are not suitable for digital mammography, because these phantoms are usually of constant thickness and are primarily sensitive to contrast limitations on film display where the image presentation cannot be changed. These limitations are easily overcome by adjustment of the display contrast at the viewing station in digital mammography.

We did find, however, that some test procedures were helpful in assessing performance. These are presented below as recommendations. Still, it is important to note that some procedures are mandatory under current regulation. It is therefore important to refer to applicable regulations that may change over time as regulators gain a better sense of how digital mammography systems perform and as the technology evolves.

WHAT FACTORS SHOULD BE TESTED IN DIGITAL MAMMOGRAPHY?

The role of many of the imaging components is identical in screen-film and digital mammography. The effects of their

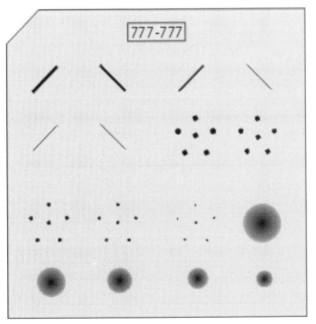

FIGURE 5-2. Schematic illustration of the structures with in the Mammographic Accreditation Phantom, introduced by the ACR and mandated by MQSA.

malfunction or maladjustment are also similar and, therefore, similar testing should be performed for these components. Such factors include the mechanical robustness of the equipment, adjustments of various positioning motions, alignment of the x-ray tube (more specifically the focal spot) with respect to the patient and the image receptor, and collimation of the x-ray beam. These tests are clearly described in documents such as the ACR Mammography Quality Control Manual (1). The frequency for such tests should be similar to those done for screen-film mammography

GENERATOR FUNCTIONS

There is another category of tests which, because of the self-testing nature of the digital system and because of technological developments in both screen-film and digital mammography, probably need not be done as frequently as now required. An example is the function of the x-ray generator. In the past 15 years, generators have become much more sophisticated and virtually all now use high-frequency power supplies. These provide precise electronic control of exposure time while being able to regulate and monitor kilovoltage and tube current during the exposure. These generators incorporate feedback and reference systems so that they are able to monitor their own performance. Once their operation has been tested in the acceptance testing of the installed system, deviations from proper performance will be rare and will generally result in the generator preventing further x-ray exposures. They generate an error code to the user suggesting the type of fault.

As part of digital mammography systems, the computer that monitors the function of the generator and other components is generally connected by Internet or telephone to the manufacturer's service department. Problems can usually be monitored remotely. With such a system, it would be reasonable to test only certain key functions and to reduce the frequency of routine comprehensive testing.

HALF VALUE LAYER

Like the kilovoltage, the half-value layer (HVL) provides a measure of the penetrating power of the x-ray beam. It should be measured periodically to ensure that there have been no changes in beam quality, possibly as a result of removal and failure to replace a beam filter when servicing the x-ray tube. In addition, knowledge of the HVL and the kilovoltage is necessary to convert measured entrance exposures to estimated mean glandular dose to the breast (mgd).

UNIFORMITY/ARTIFACTS

The flat-field corrections performed in the preliminary processing of digital mammograms should produce images that are uniform in intensity without artifacts. The sensitivity of individual detector elements can drift over time, and the calibration maps may have to be remeasured. Therefore, it is important to test the system for uniformity. This can be accomplished by periodically imaging a uniform slab of plastic (polymethylmethacrylate). It is best if this measurement is performed with a different radiation intensity from that used for the actual calibration. This can be done by employing a slab of a different thickness. This would make the test sensitive to any nonlinearity that may be present in the detector response to radiation.

At the same time as this test is performed, it is useful to image a small (e.g., 1-cm diameter, 1-mm thick) disk placed on the plastic slab. This allows a measurement of contrast between regions-of-interest (ROIs) on the image of the disk and on a similar area of the background adjacent to the disk. The standard deviation of the pixel values can be used as an index of noise and a practical signal-difference-to-noise ratio (SDNR) can be defined as:

$$SDNR = (Q_{out} - Q_{in}/(\sigma^2_{out} + \sigma^2_{in})^{1/2}$$

where Q_{out} and Q_{in} are the mean pixel values in the two ROIs and σ_{in} and σ_{out} are the standard deviations about the mean in each ROI. One of the desirable features of digital mammography is that software can be created to analyze the image and calculate this value automatically, thus saving effort and reducing the measurement variability introduced by human error.

DOSE VERSUS SIGNAL AND LINEARITY

One of the great potential advantages of digital mammography arises from the decoupling of image acquisition and display. This allows flexible adjustment of image brightness and contrast and even permits enhancement of sharpness. It also presents a potential danger in that an image can be made to look reasonably good over a widely varying range of radiation exposure. If too low an exposure is used, the image SNR will suffer. On the other hand, if the dose is too high, the image quality will usually appear to be excellent, but the dose to the breast will be excessive. Unless the relationship between the radiation exposure or dose and the pixel signal value in the digitized image is known and monitored, this can easily occur without the operator being aware of it. Therefore, it is important to measure this relationship on the equipment. This is easy to do because the data are already in quantitative form. In

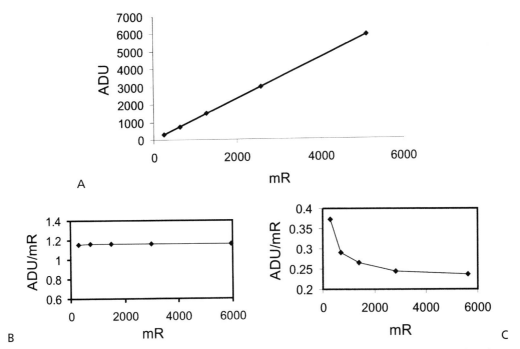

FIGURE 5-3. Sensitivity calibration of the digital system. **(A)** pixel value in analog-to-digital units (ADU) vs. exposure or mAs. **(B)** Evaluation of linearity. Slope of the curve in **(A)** is shown at each exposure for a highly linear system. **(C)** Results for a system with poor linearity.

the experiment, whose results are illustrated in Figure 5-3A, the mA or mAs is varied for a series of exposures. The exposure[1] of the x-ray system at the entrance surface to a breast of specified compressed thickness (e.g., 4.5 cm) is measured with a dosimeter and the pixel value in an ROI is plotted versus exposure. Figure 5-3A also illustrates the linearity of detector response; however, a more sensitive method of evaluating the linearity of the system is illustrated in Figure 5-3B and 5-3C. Alternatively, a linear regression can be performed on the data and the deviation from the linear fit is plotted.

Experiments like those of Figure 5-3 are performed for each kV and target/filter combination of the system. The exposure output in milliroentgens/mAs can be calculated, so that the entrance exposure can be calculated for any kV and mAs. From the exposure, kV, and HVL, the dose (mgd) is calculated using tables available in the literature (2).

NOISE VERSUS DOSE

As discussed in Chapter 2, the dominant source of noise in the digital image should be due to quantum statistics.

Therefore, for an ROI in the image, after correction for a "dark signal" has been performed (see Chapter 3), the standard deviation of the pixel value about its mean in the ROI should be proportional to the square root of the mean pixel value. Alternatively, the variance (standard deviation squared) should be directly proportional to the mean pixel value and the line (Fig. 5-4) should ideally pass through the origin of the graph. This would imply that with no x-rays, there is no noise. In reality the intercept is nonzero, and the value of the variance for no x-ray exposure provides a measure of the system noise because of amplifiers and other electronic sources, as well as structural (fixed pattern) noise that has not adequately been removed in the detector correction process (see Chapter 3). This could be the result of nonlinearity of detector response or temporal changes in the detector between calibrations.

It is also possible for the relationship to be nonlinear, indicating that there are also sources of signal dependent noise that are not the result of simple quantum fluctuation. These were discussed briefly in Chapter 3.

SPATIAL RESOLUTION

In screen-film mammography, spatial resolution of high-contrast structures is usually limited by the combination of focal spot size and magnification, not by the image receptor, because current screen-film products have reso-

---

[1]Exposure and its unit, the roentgen, is no longer an accepted quantity according to the Système Internationale (SI) system of units. The currently accepted quantity is air kerma, and its unit is Joules/kg of air. Nevertheless, the roentgen is still in common use in North America.

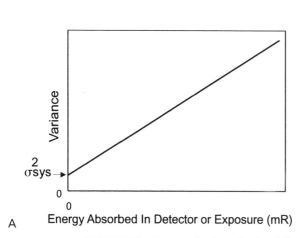

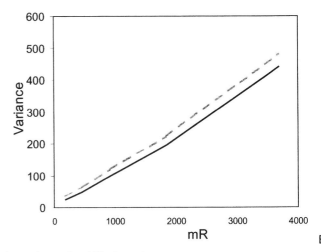

FIGURE 5-4. Characterization of noise. **(A)** Noise variance should be linearly related to the number of quanta used to produce the image, which is in turn related to the exposure or energy absorbed by the detector. The intercept provides an estimate of the system's electronic noise. **(B)** Actual experimental data showing slight variation with position.

lutions above 20 lp/mm. In digital mammography, the size of the dels in the detector is generally the limiting factor, and the limiting spatial resolution (that which would be measured with a lead bar pattern) is generally lower. Limiting resolution is not a very useful measure as it only describes the finest very high-contrast details that could be imaged. Such high-contrast structures are not present in the breast. With the quantitative data available in digital mammography, it is possible to do a much more sophisticated test of resolution very easily in terms of the modulation transfer function (MTF). The MTF describes, for each level of detail, the efficiency of the imaging system at transferring the inherent subject contrast to the output. In the DMIST trial, a simple test tool for measuring MTF (Fig. 5-5) was introduced. This consists of a square of aluminum with a smaller square of a more highly, but still only partially attenuating material, affixed to it. Its sides form a slight angle with respect to those of the larger sheet. To measure MTF, the tool is placed on the tabletop or at a fixed distance above it and imaged. Using a software tool whose user interface is illustrated in Figure 5-6, the profiles of x-ray transmission of the pattern are measured from the digital image. The MTF can then be calculated. An example is shown in Figure 5-7, where it is seen that the MTF is different in different directions in the images, thereby suggesting a directional dependence of detector resolution.

ARTIFACTS

Nonuniformities due to drifts in the flat-field correction were mentioned earlier. Other artifacts can occur because of detector malfunctions causing "dead pixels" or dead rows or columns in the image. It is also possible, particularly for systems where the image must be pieced or "stitched" together from subimages, that there can be distortions where these images abut one another. A tool for testing for such distortions is shown in Figure 5-8. Examples of a relatively artifact-free system and one exhibiting a stitching error are given in Figure 5-9. This test will identify problems that can occur in systems which involve scanning the detector or a readout laser beam. Speed irregularity in mechanical scanning or nonuniform motion or jitter in laser alignment can seriously reduce MTF in one direction or cause other artifacts.

FIGURE 5-5. Test tool for measuring MTF.

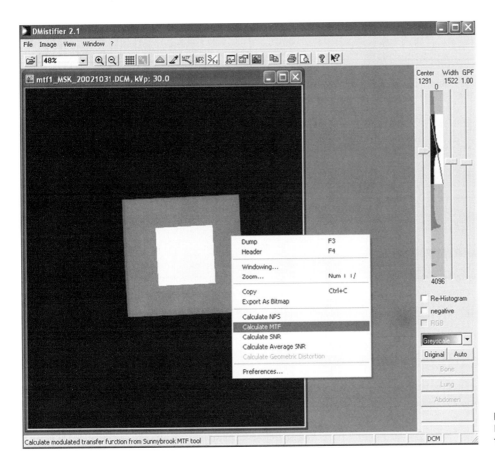

FIGURE 5-6. User interface for DMISTIFIER image analysis software to calculate MTF.

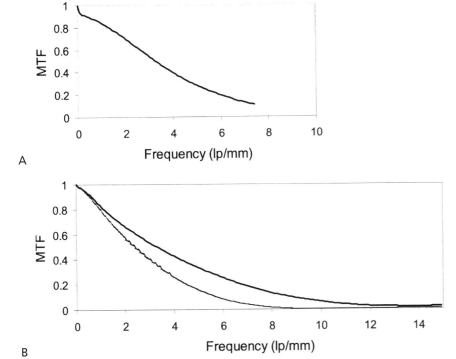

A

B

FIGURE 5-7. Measured MTFs of digital systems. **(A)** 100 μm dels, MTF similar for all four edges of test pattern. **(B)** 50 μm del scanning system with maladjustment of scan speed. MTF differs in slot and scanning directions.

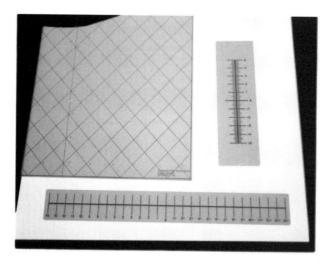

FIGURE 5-8. Tool for measuring image geometric distortion.

QUALITY CONTROL FOR IMAGE DISPLAY

Display is a critical component of the imaging process in digital mammography. For both softcopy and hardcopy display, it is important that both the monitor(s) and printer are calibrated to the DICOM grayscale standard display function (NEMA), as it provides consistency in the way contrast is presented to the viewer (3)

Softcopy Display

For softcopy display, it is important to verify that the monitors have been set up properly and provide adequate brightness and contrast over their entire dynamic range. To do this effectively, it is necessary to display a standard pattern on the monitors and to perform photometric measurements of brightness and contrast. It is also important to test the resolution of the device to ensure that its electronic focus is properly adjusted. The most commonly used pattern was developed by the Society of Motion Picture and Television Engineers (SMPTE) and has been used on analog systems for many years (4) (Fig. 5-10).

For digital mammography, DICOM versions of the SMPTE pattern can be created, stored on the digital mammography system computer, and displayed whenever the tests are to be performed. The pattern has tests of spatial resolution and contrast scale to allow testing the display to ensure that it provides its maximum possible dynamic range. For example, the display should be set to allow visualization of transitions both between 0% and 5% of full scale and between 95% and 100% of full scale on the monitor simultaneously (Fig. 5-11). Computer programs are available that generate an SMPTE image of arbitrary size in DICOM file format (3). The American Association of Physicists in Medicine has established a Task Group (TG-18 Assessment of Display Performance for Medical Imaging Systems), which has developed a number of test procedures for this purpose (5,6).

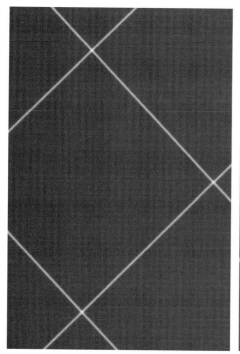

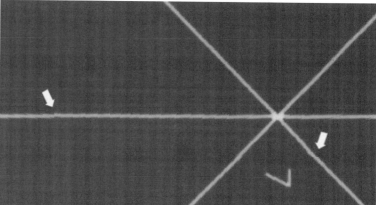

A   B

FIGURE 5-9. (A) Image of the distortion tool obtained on a system without discernible distortion. **(B)** Example of a distortion artifact caused by "stitching" subimages together. Arrows indicate discontinuities.

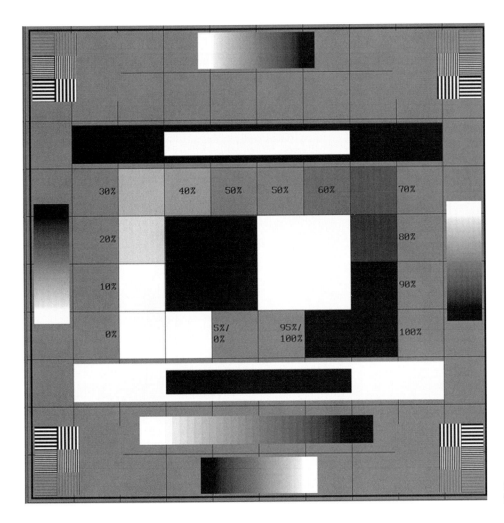

FIGURE 5-10. The SMPTE display test pattern.

Hardcopy Display

Evaluation of performance of the hardcopy display device is similar to that for softcopy. The hardcopy device is generally a laser film printer using either conventional film chemistry or dry processing. Dry systems often have self-tests incorporated in the printer that correct for drifts in sensitometry. For wet processing systems, adequate attention must be given to the film processor, using sensitometry and densitometry techniques as employed in screen-film mammography.

For testing, a SMPTE image can be generated digitally in the printer or can be sent from the digital mammography system.

CONCLUSION

Quality control for screen-film mammography is a mature activity, consisting of a well-established system of tests enshrined by law in the United States. For digital mam-

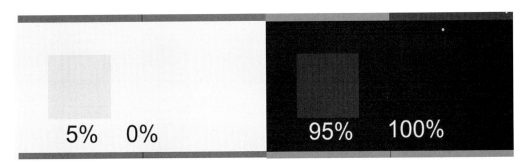

FIGURE 5-11. The 0%-5% and 95%-100% transitions that should be visible when the display is properly set up.

mography, we currently have a reasonable idea of the types of functions that require testing, but the optimum test procedures, the tolerance limits for measurements, and the required testing frequency have not yet been optimized. As we gain more practical experience with digital mammography, QC procedures will evolve. Likely, many of these will be automated, greatly reducing the time and cost of quality control.

REFERENCES

1. Hendrick RE, Bassett LW, Botsco MA, et al. ACR Mammography Quality Control Manual. Reston, VA: American College of Radiology; 1999.

2. Dance DR, Skinner CL, Young KC, et al. Additional factors for the estimation of mean glandular breast dose using the UK mammography dosimetry protocol. Phys Med Biol 2000;45:3225–3240.

3. NEMA. Digital Imaging and Communications in Medicine (DICOM). Part 14: Grayscale Standard Display Function (PS 3.14-2001). National Electrical Manufacturers Association, Rosslyn, Virginia.

4. SMPTE. RP133 Specifications for Medical Diagnostic Imaging Test Pattern for Television Monitors and Hardcopy Recording Cameras. White Plains, NY: Society of Motion Picture and Television Engineers.

5. Clunie D. DICOM toolkit http://www.dclunie.com/dicom3tools.html accessed on 1/6/2003.

6. American Association of Physicists in Medicine (AAMP) Task Group #18. Assessment of display performance of medical imaging systems. Version 9.0http://deckard.mc.duke.edu/samei/tg18, accessed 1/10/2003.

6

COMPUTER-AIDED DETECTION IN DIGITAL MAMMOGRAPHY

ROBERT M. NISHIKAWA

INTRODUCTION

Two of the most promising technologies for improving the earlier detection of breast cancer are full-field digital mammography (FFDM) and computer-aided diagnosis (CAD) (1). Computer-aided diagnosis is defined as a diagnosis made by a radiologist who considers the output of a computer analysis of the image when making his or her interpretation. While the development of these two technologies has been to date independent, there is a natural synergy between them. The acquisition of mammograms in digital form, without the intermediate steps of recording the image on film and then digitizing the film, should result in a very powerful approach to improving the detection of breast cancer. This chapter provides a brief overview of the state-of-the-art in CAD development and then describes the complementary strengths of CAD and FFDM when combined clinically. Finally, current research and the challenges ahead for CAD and FFDM will be discussed.

STATE-OF-THE-ART IN COMPUTER-AIDED DIAGNOSIS

Throughout the 1990s, research in computer-aided diagnosis (CAD) for mammography had grown rapidly. There are two main areas of interest: techniques for the automated detection of breast lesions and techniques for the classification of breast lesions as benign or malignant. Detection schemes are slightly more developed with three commercial systems being available in the United States. Detection schemes are capable of detecting approximately 80% to 90% of breast cancers present on mammograms at a false–positive rate of 0.1–1.0 per image. Classification

schemes are capable of performing at levels comparable to or exceeding those of radiologists.

Evidence is accumulating that when implemented clinically, CAD will improve radiologists' performance in reading screening mammograms. At least four studies have shown that automated detection schemes can detect breast cancer on mammograms that were called normal by a radiologist (2–5). Two studies have shown, in simulated clinical reading situations, that CAD can improve radiologists' ability to detect breast lesions (6,7). Freer and Ulissey (8) found in a one-year period (12,860 patients) that CAD increased the number of cancers detected by 19.5%—eight additional cancers out of 49 were detected when the radiologist was aided by the computer. This was at the cost of increasing the recall rate from 6.5% to 7.7%. Of the 986 recalls, 156 were from the CAD reading. More clinical studies like this one are needed to understand fully the advantages and disadvantages of CAD.

Evidence for the benefits of computer classification schemes comes from three observer studies that showed radiologists' performance improved significantly when they were assisted by the computer classifier (9–12). Sensitivities above 90% with a positive-predictive value of approximately 60% have been achieved. This is compared to radiologists who typically have 85% sensitivity and positive-predictive values of approximately 30%.

SYNERGISM BETWEEN COMPUTER-AIDED DIAGNOSIS AND FULL-FIELD DIGITAL MAMMOGRAPHY

While the development of FFDM and CAD have been, for the most part, independent, it is likely that for either system to gain wide clinical acceptance they will have to be sold together as a package. This is because there are serious limitations to each when operating without the other in terms of cost, logistics of use, display, archiving, and accuracy.

Robert M. Nishikawa is a shareholder in R2 Technology, Inc. (Los Altos, CA). It is the University of Chicago Conflict of Interest Policy that investigators disclose publicly actual or potential significant financial interests, which may appear to be affected by the research activities.

Cost of the Systems

Because of its high cost—estimated to be between $300,000 and $500,000—FFDM needs to offer radiologists more than just better image quality for dense breasts. In a similar vein, while implementation of CAD using film digitizing and film viewing is feasible, it will increase the time technologists and radiologists need to perform their work. CAD on an FFDM system would offer radiologists enhanced display features and automated second opinions, and the added CAD component would be transparent to the technologist. Furthermore, the cost for a CAD system using film digitization is approximately $150,000. A large component of that cost is the film digitizer, which has a retail price of approximately $30,000. In addition, given that most FFDM systems have at least one medium-to-high-end workstation, a packaged system of FFDM and CAD would be significantly cheaper than buying the two components separately. It is nearly as easy as adding CAD software to the existing FFDM system.

Clinical Implementation

Currently CAD can be performed using screen-film mammograms, but the process can be simplified if FFDM were used (see Fig. 6–1). To implement CAD using screen-film

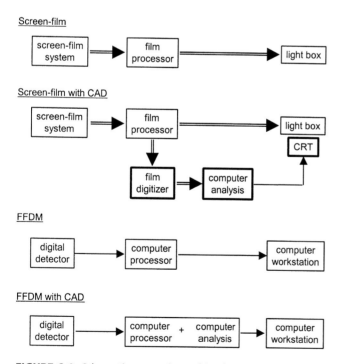

FIGURE 6-1. Schematic comparison of implementing CAD using screen-film mammography vs. using full-field digital mammography (FFDM) with softcopy reading. An arrow with a single line indicates an automated task and an arrow with a double line indicates a technologist-mediated task. Boxes with thick lines indicate additional hardware compared to a system without CAD.

images requires that the technologist digitize the films before the films are hung on a light box or film alternator. Further, either the computer output needs to be printed on film, which would require the films to be manually hung on the light box with the mammograms, or displayed on a CRT monitor, which needs to be situated near the light box. If CAD were to be implemented with a FFDM system using softcopy reading, then the process can be completely automated, so that there would be no additional human intervention involved. Obviously from a workflow point of view, CAD implemented with FFDM is more efficient. CAD implemented using screen-film mammography would require, at a minimum, additional technologist time.

While it may seem somewhat trivial, it is necessary for the CAD program to communicate with the rest of the world, that is, with the Picture Archiving and Communication System (PACS), the display workstation, and so on. DICOM supplement 50 is a standard for mammography CAD structure reporting class. This standard allows the results of the computer analysis to be stored with the image. The display workstation can then be instructed to take the stored information and place it as an overlay on the digital mammogram that indicates the computer output.

Quality of Digitized Screen-Film Mammograms

From a scientific point of view, the real excitement of applying CAD to digital mammograms is the possibility of significantly improved performance of the CAD schemes. The advantages of FFDM over screen-film mammography are well documented (as discussed in Chapter 2). They include wider latitude, lower noise, and higher signal-to-noise ratio (SNR). The advantages of FFDM over digitized screen-film mammography are even greater. Film digitizers, while fairly linear, have a dynamic range that is smaller than screen-film systems, which have a maximum optical density of greater than 4.0. Furthermore, film digitizers add noise to the image, particularly in dark regions of the images. Compared to a digitized mammogram, one would expect that a FFDM image to have better SNR at low exposures, because film granularity is a significant noise component in a screen-film image (13–15). Similarly, because of the added noise of the digitizer, the FFDM image should have better SNR than a digitized mammogram at high exposures. At intermediate exposures, FFDM systems produce images of higher SNR, because FFDM systems have better quantum detection efficiency than screen-film systems (16). With better SNR, it should be possible to extract information from the image that is more accurate and thereby improve the computer's ability to discriminate between true and false lesions and/or between benign and malignant lesions.

Softcopy Reading versus Hardcopy Reading

The display of computer detection results to the radiologist is awkward with screen-film systems. Either a hardcopy (paper or film) output must be printed—which has to be put in the patient jacket and be available to the radiologist to view—or a softcopy monitor must be placed near the viewing station or be built into the viewing station. Either method requires that the radiologist look away from the films to view the computer results and then look back at the films. While this seems rather trivial, it can become bothersome for the radiologist and could, therefore, reduce the radiologist's productivity and accuracy. A softcopy display for the digital mammograms (in place of film), where the computer detections can be turned on and off, would permit a very efficient means for conveying the computer results to the radiologist.

To obtain the maximum potential of FFDM, images should be processed to enhance the visibility of abnormalities. As discussed in Chapter 7, different types of lesions need different types of enhancement (17). To implement multiple-processing algorithms, a softcopy display is needed. However, viewing digital mammograms on softcopy has not been perfected. There are a number of technical problems involving speed of display and ease of use. These will be remedied with more research and evolving technology. It is still unproven, however, that the accuracy of softcopy reading is comparable to reading film mammograms. With the use of CAD, however, performance of softcopy reading could exceed reading of hardcopy films alone.

CAD could help solve one of the major problems with displaying a digital mammogram on a CRT monitor. To see the fine detail of the image, all pixels in the image would need to be displayed. This is extremely difficult or not possible, especially for systems with a pixel size of less than 100 μ or when trying to display an image of a large breast. However, with computer detection algorithms reaching up to 98% sensitivity for clustered calcifications, one could display the full image at lower resolution to search for masses, architectural distortions, and so on, and rely on the computer to locate clustered calcifications. The radiologist would only have to zoom areas where the computer identified a cluster, instead of panning through the full image at full resolution.

Image Archiving

A single digital mammogram is between 10 and 60 Mbytes in size. A four-view exam then is between 40 and 240 Mbytes. Furthermore, for women with large breasts, more than one exposure is needed to image all portions of the breast. In extreme cases, this can mean as many as 20 exposures. For a screening center that performs 10,000 exams each year, the storage requirements, assuming only four images per patient, is between 400 and 2400 GBytes. Since by law, mammograms need to be kept indefinitely (until the patient dies), the storage requirements for digital mammography are enormous. The commercial storage solutions are relatively expensive when compared to the cost of the FFDM system.

Image compression is one possible solution to this problem. However, using lossless compression gives only modest amounts of compression, that is, approximately 2:1 or 3:1. There is reluctance to using lossy compression, because it is felt that some information may be lost or distorted in a decompressed image that could affect the diagnosis. A novel approach to this problem is to use content-based compression (18). In this technique, areas of the breast that contain significant diagnostic information are compressed losslessly and all other areas of the breast are compressed lossy. In this way, compression ratios of greater than 10:1 can be obtained without compromising the correct diagnosis. Computer-aided diagnosis schemes can be used to identify the regions in the image that should undergo lossless compression. Current detection schemes do not have 100% sensitivity, so there is still a risk that important diagnostic information could be lost. However, it is possible to tune a CAD scheme so that the sensitivity increases, at the cost of higher false–positive rate. Because the results of the computer detection scheme are not being used by radiologists in this application, the high false–positive rate is not a problem, although it will reduce the final overall compression ratio to which the image is finally compressed. It is also likely, as more companies develop a product, that the accuracy of CAD schemes will improve and, as a result, content-based compression will become more feasible.

Quantitative Analyses

One must be somewhat daring to do quantitative analysis using a screen-film system because one needs to know fairly accurately the characteristic curve of that system. While it is straightforward to make such a measurement, the characteristic curve depends upon the film processing conditions (e.g., the nature of the chemistry and the developer temperature). These conditions will vary over time during the day and, therefore, short of calibrating the film processor for every film, it is not possible to know the exact characteristic curve of the screen-film system. Digital systems have stable characteristic curves, so that one measurement a day is sufficient to determine accurately the characteristic curve for any image taken on a particular machine. Currently there are CAD schemes that try to estimate the thickness of objects based on the film density (19,20) and also that try to transform the image based on the noise in the image (21). Both of these are subject to error caused by variation in the film processing conditions. With a digital system, very accurate estimates of object thickness and noise properties can be made

AREAS OF RESEARCH

CAD Using Digitized Film versus Digital Mammograms

An important question is whether CAD schemes have higher performance when operating on digital images from an FFDM system then when operating on digitized screen-film images, as one might postulate. This will require a large database of mammograms from a set of women who have been imaged on both screen-film and FFDM systems. Actually, one of the hurdles in the development of CAD for FFDM systems will be the lack of cases from women who have cancer. These cases are needed to optimize the different CAD techniques.

Commercial systems for automated detection are robust and accurate because of the large databases of digitized screen-film mammograms that were developed. Between 1,000 and 2,000 cancer cases were used to design, train, and evaluate the commercial systems. In North America, there may be only a few hundred FFDM cases currently available where a cancer is visible, and some of these were acquired on out-dated systems (e.g., prototype models). Clearly, the lack of images will severely hamper efforts to develop a robust and accurate CAD system for FFDM. Because of a lack of images, there is very little in the literature on CAD applied to FFDM. Nawano et al. have a database of 4,148 digital mammograms including 267 cases of breast cancer (22). These were acquired using a Fuji Computed Radiography 9000 system. They were able to obtain sensitivities of 89.9% for masses and 92.8% for clustered calcifications, at false–positive rates of 1.35 false masses per image and 0.40 false clusters per image.

It may not be necessary, however, to have a thousand cancer cases. It may be possible to use the knowledge gained on digitized screen-film systems to guide the optimization of FFDM-based systems. For example, if one can determine the differences in features, such as contrast, between digital and digitized images, then one could predict how to modify the digitized-film-based scheme to work on FFDM images. Furthermore, for clustered calcifications, where there are multiple calcifications per cluster, partial optimization can be done on a hundred images, which could contain over a thousand calcifications.

Recently, General Electric (GE) Medical Systems received FDA clearance to market in the United States computer-aided detection schemes on its FFDM system. The CAD schemes were developed by R2 Technology, Inc. (Los Altos, CA) specifically for the GE FFDM images. In a preliminary study (23), the R2 system detected 84% of masses and 97% of clustered classification with 0.5 false detection

per image for each CAD scheme ref. These results are comparable to those obtained on digitized screen-film mammograms except that the false–positive rate for microcalcifications was higher on the FFDM images. It should be noted, however, that FFDM images came from a different set of patients than the film mammograms.

Pixel Size and CAD Performance

Several fundamental questions that remain to be answered are common between CAD and FFDM. These include optimum pixel size, best technique to implement the systems clinically, and clinical efficacy.

Prototype and commercially available FFDM systems that are currently in clinical use or evaluation range in pixel size by a factor of 2.5–40 μ to 100 μ. While it seems at first thought that smaller pixels would be better, there are drawbacks to using smaller pixels. First, display monitors can now only display images that are approximately 2,048 by 2,560, which corresponds to a digital mammogram with 100-μ pixel size. It is not possible to display the full image at full resolution for a smaller pixel size. Also the size of the image is inversely proportional to the square of the pixel size. Large image size reduces acquisition and display speeds and puts a larger burden on storage requirements. These drawbacks are secondary to producing diagnostic images. It is unclear at this time what the appropriate pixel size should be.

Intuitively, since fine structure, such as spiculations emanating from a mass, has diagnostic relevance, an FFDM system needs high spatial resolution. However, a digital image can be processed after it has been acquired to enhance high spatial frequencies, and thereby preferentially increase the contrast of small objects, such as microcalcifications. The drawback to enhancing the microcalcifications is that the noise will also be enhanced, so that the net overall effect presenting as microcalcifications may be to camouflage cancers with image noise. It is more important, then, to compare the signal-to-noise ratios (SNRs) for different size objects, if one wants to compare the effect of pixel size on detectability of small objects. The SNR, as the name implies, depends on both the signal (i.e., contrast) and the noise properties of the system.

To illustrate the importance of SNR over spatial resolution, one only has to compare FFDM systems to screen-film systems. A mammographic screen-film system has a limiting resolution of more than 20 cycles/mm. FFDM have limiting resolution of between 5 and 10 cycles/mm. Yet smaller objects are visible in FFDM images of test objects than in screen-film images (24).

Similarly, the appropriate pixel size for digitizing an image to subject it to CAD schemes is not known. Two separate studies by Chan and colleagues give somewhat surprising results. For their scheme to detect individual microcalcifications, the performance improved as the pixel size decreased from 140 to 35 μ (25). However, for classifying microcalcifications as benign or malignant, the scheme's performance did not improve as the pixel size decreased from 100 μ down to 35 μ (26). Most radiologists and medical physicists argue that higher spatial resolution is needed in screening mammography because the presence of a calcification can be seen at somewhat "coarse" resolution, but fine detail and, therefore high spatial resolution, are needed to distinguish benign from malignant calcifications for diagnostic mammography.

This author interprets this paradox as follows. For a computer to distinguish an actual calcification from a computer detected false-positive, high spatial resolution is needed because, for the computer, fine detail is necessary to distinguish an actual calcification from, for example, a film artifact on a digitized image. To distinguish benign from malignant calcifications, the relevant shape factor is whether the calcifications are linear or branching and this can be done at 100-μ pixel resolution. The exact shape of calcifications is not diagnostic, because the SNR of the image is insufficient to determine accurately the precise shape or border of small calcifications. Evidence to support this assertion comes from an observer study conducted by Jiang et al. (11). They had 10 radiologists rating the likelihood that calcifications were malignant and whether they would recommend that the patient have a biopsy. The radiologists read the original mammograms: the four standard views and two spot-magnification views. A computer analyzed only the standard view mammograms digitized at 100-μ pixel resolution. As can be seen in Table 6–1, the computer outperformed the radiologists in terms of area under the ROC curve, sensitivity, and specificity. Furthermore Chan et al. also conducted an observer study asking radiologists to read clusters extracted from digitized mammograms (27). They found no significant difference in radiologists' performance in classifying the clusters.

Thus, this author concludes that 100-μ pixel size is sufficient for digital mammography, if the system has high detective quantum efficiency (DQE) at intermediate spatial frequencies (approximately 1–3 cycles/mm). In many digital systems, this can only be obtained by having a small pixel size, but newer so-called direct digital detectors can achieve this goal with 100-μ pixel size, at least in theory (28).

Impact of CAD/FFDM on Radiologists' Performance

Evidence is accumulating that CAD can improve radiologists' performance, at least in simulated clinical situations. These are for the cases where radiologists are reading screen-film mammograms and computer algorithms are operating on digitized film mammograms. While the same is probably true for radiologists reading FFDM images and the computer operating on FFDM images, it remains to be proven. It is possible that both the computer and the radiologist perform better using FFDM images, but the improvement by the radiologist is such that the added value of CAD is small. If the image quality of FFDM were so great that radiologists could clearly see all cancers, even those in dense tissue, then CAD would have limited value since radiologists would not miss many cancers. However, initial studies indicate that this is not true for the present generation of digital systems (29).

The observer study of CAD applied to FFDM was by Nawano et al. (22). They used ROC analysis on data collected from five radiologists reading using 344 mammograms from 86 women. They found that the average area under the ROC curve increased by a statistically significant amount (p <0.022) when the radiologists used the computer aid.

SUMMARY

Both computer-aided diagnosis and full field digital mammography systems are beginning to undergo clinical evaluation. The development of these two fields has taken place in parallel and nearly independently until recently. There is a strong synergism between the two. Limitations of one system can be overcome or partially compensated by the strengths of the other system. In addition, FFDM will facilitate quantitative image analysis that will open new avenues in CAD research. The most important question still

TABLE 6-1. COMPARISON OF RADIOLOGISTS AND COMPUTER IN CLASSIFYING CALCIFICATIONS AS BENIGN OR MALIGNANT. THE RADIOLOGISTS READ THE ORIGINAL STANDARD AND MAGNIFICATION VIEWS. THE COMPUTER ANALYZED ONLY THE STANDARD VIEWS DIGITIZED AT 100-μ PIXEL RESOLUTION. A$_Z$ IS THE AREA UNDER THE ROC (RECEIVER OPERATING CHARACTERISTIC) CURVE.

	A$_Z$	Sensitivity	Specificity
Radiologists using standard views and spot magnification views	0.61	74%	32%
Computer using only standard views digitized at 100 μ	0.80	90%	50%

remains whether CAD implemented on an FFDM system can improve radiologists' performance in detecting and diagnosing breast cancer.

REFERENCES

1. Shtern F. Digital mammography and related technologies: A perspective from the National Cancer Institute. Radiology 1992; 183:629–630.
2. Schmidt RA, Nishikawa RM, Osnis R, et al. Computerized detection of lesions missed by mammography. In: Doi K, Giger ML, Nishikawa RM, et al., eds. Digital Mammography '96. Amsterdam: Elsevier Science, 1996;105–110.
3. te Brake GM, Karssemeijer N, Hendriks JHCL. Automated detection of breast carcinomas not detected in a screening program. Radiology 1998;207:465–471.
4. Warren Burhenne LJ, Wood SA, D'Orsi CJ, et al. Potential contribution of computer-aided detection to the sensitivity of screening mammography. Radiology 2000;215:554–562.
5. Moberg K, Bjurstam N, Wilczek B, et al. Computer assisted detection of interval breast cancers. Eur J Radiol 2001;39:104–110.
6. Chan H-P, Doi K, Vyborny CJ, et al. Improvement in radiologists' detection of clustered microcalcifications on mammograms: The potential of computer-aided diagnosis. Invest Radiol 1990; 25:1102–1110.
7. Kegelmeyer WP, Pruneda JM, Bourland PD, et al. Computer-aided mammographic screening for spiculated lesions. Radiology 1994;191:331–337.
8. Freer TW, Ulissey MJ. Screening mammography with computer-aided detection: Prospective study of 12,860 patients in a community breast center. Radiology 2001;220:781–786.
9. Getty DJ, Pickett RM, D'Orsi CJ, et al. Enhanced interpretation of diagnostic images. Invest Radiol 1988;23:240–252.
10. Chan HP, Sahiner B, Helvie MA, et al. Improvement of radiologists' characterization of mammographic masses by using computer-aided diagnosis: An ROC study. Radiology 1999;212: 817–827.
11. Jiang Y, Nishikawa RM, Schmidt RA, et al. Improving breast cancer diagnosis with computer-aided diagnosis. Acad Radiol 1999;6:22–33.
12. Huo Z, Giger M, Vyborny C. Analysis of computer-aided diagnosis on radiologists' performance using an independent database. Proc SPIE 2001;4324:41–51.
13. Bunch PC, Huff KE, Van Metter R. Analysis of the detective quantum efficiency of a radiographic film-screen combination. J Opt Soc Am A 1987;4:902–909.
14. Chakraborty DP, Barnes GT. Radiographic mottle and patient exposure in mammography. Radiology 1982;145:815–821.
15. Nishikawa RM, Yaffe MJ. Signal-to-noise properties of mammographic film-screen systems. Med Phys 1985;12:32–39.
16. Vedantham S, Karellas A, Suryanarayanan S, et al. Full breast digital mammography with an amorphous silicon-based flat panel detector: Physical characteristics of a clinical prototype. Med Phys 2000;27:558–567.
17. Pisano ED, Cole EB, Major S, et al. Radiologist Preferences for Digital Mammography Display. Radiology 2000;216:820–830.
18. Grinstead B, Sari-Sarraf H, Gleason S, et al. Preliminary validation of content-based compression of mammographic images. Proc SPIE 2001;4322:1179–1190.
19. Highnam R, Brady M, English R. Detecting film-screen artifacts in mammography using a model-based approach. IEEE Trans Med Imaging 1999;18:1016–1024.
20. Jiang Y, Nishikawa RM, Giger ML, et al. Method of extracting microcalcifications' signal area and signal thickness from digital mammograms. Proc SPIE 1992;1778:28–36.
21. Karssemeijer N. Adaptive noise equalization and recognition of microcalcification clusters in mammograms. Int J Pattern Recognition Artificial Intelligence 1993;7:1357–1376.
22. Nawano S, Murakami K, Moriyama N, et al. Computer-aided diagnosis in full digital mammography. Invest Radiol 1999;34: 310–316.
23. O'Shaughnessy K, Castellino R, Muller S, et al. Computer Aided Detection (CAD) on 90 Biopsy-Proven Breast Cancer Cases acquired on a Full Field Digital Mammography (FFDM) System. Radiology 2001;221(P):471.
24. Nishikawa RM, Mawdsley GE, Fenster A, et al. Scanned-projection digital mammography. Medical Physics 1987;14:717–727.
25. Chan H-P, Niklason LT, Ikeda DM, et al. Digitization requirements in mammography: Effects on computer-aided detection of microcalcifications. Medical Physics 1994;21:1203–1211.
26. Chan H-P, Sahiner B, Petrick N, et al. Effects of pixel size on classification of microcalcifications on digitized mammograms. Proc SPIE 1996;2710:30–41.
27. Chan HP, Helvie MA, Petrick N, et al. Digital mammography: Observer performance study of the effects of pixel size on the characterization of malignant and benign microcalcifications. Academic Radiology 2001;8:454–466.
28. Rowlands JA, Yorkston J. Flat panel detectors for digital radiography. In: Beutel J, Kundel H, Van Metter R, eds. Handbook of Medical Imaging. Bellingham, WA: SPIE, 2000;223-328.
29. Lewin JM, Hendrick RE, D'Orsi CJ, et al. Comparison of full-field digital mammography with screen-film mammography for cancer detection: Results of 4,945 paired examinations. Radiology 2001;218:873–880.

7

IMAGE PROCESSING

ETTA D. PISANO

Image processing is critical for the success of digital mammography, as it is for the success of all projection radiographic imaging systems. In addition, mammography requires specific processing to achieve images suitable for the different mammography reading purposes. Recent results of a preference study suggest that different presentation formats are appropriate for different clinical tasks (screening vs. diagnosis) and for the diagnosis of different lesion types (calcifications vs. masses). In addition, the type of image processing preferred by radiologists differed by machine type (Fischer Medical Imaging, Denver, Colorado, General Electric Medical Systems, Milwaukee, Wisconsin, Trex, a division of Hologic, Inc., Bedford, Mass) (1).

The study utilized 28 digital mammograms obtained on Fischer, General Electric (GE), and Trex devices. Most of the cases used had mammographic lesions that had undergone biopsy, and all had at least one mammographic finding that was presumed benign by virtue of stability since prior mammograms. Twelve radiologists reviewed eight different processed versions of these same cases and ranked the images relative to the accompanying screen-film mammograms for their ability to depict the features of the lesion that best revealed the known diagnosis. The algorithms studied were Manual Intensity Windowing (MIW), Histogram-based Intensity Windowing (HIW), Mixture-Model Intensity Windowing (MMIW), Contrast Limited Adaptive Histogram Equalization (CLAHE), MUSICA (Agfa®), Unsharp Masking (UM), Peripheral Equalization (PE) and Trex® processing. These choices were based partially on preliminary laboratory studies (2–6). Of course, all potentially useful algorithms could not be included in this study. Each of the algorithms included in this study is described in detail below.

INTENSITY WINDOWING ALGORITHMS (IW)

Through the application of intensity windowing algorithms, readers select a small portion of the full intensity range of an image and then remap those values to the full intensity range of the display device. This should allow for the selection of specific intensity values of interest in a particular image. But, the values must be chosen carefully to increase the contrast between features of interest, as, for example, cancer calcifications against a dense mammographic background. The three versions of IW that were explored in the International Digital Mammography Development Group (IDMDG) study were MIW, HIW, and MMIW. These algorithms differ only in how intensity values of interest are selected.

Manual Intensity Windowing

Manual Intensity Windowing (MIW) can be performed by an expert mammography technologist or radiologist who interactively adjusts the contrast levels as appropriate for each image. Often, the goal of windowing with this algorithm is to manually reproduce the appearance of a screen-film mammogram, or to "see through" the densest areas of the breast optimally.

Histogram-based Intensity Windowing

Histogram-based intensity windowing (HIW) allows the computer to automatically window the image by examining the histogram of intensity values of the digital image to automatically identify regions of interest. For example, the skin and densest parts of the breast provide specifically identifiable portions of the image intensity histogram and can be displayed with specific windowing unique to them once the computer evaluates the histogram.

Mixture-Model Intensity Windowing

Mixture-Model Intensity Windowing (MMIW) allows segmentation of the parts of the mammogram, that is, dense versus fatty components, using a combination of geometric and statistical techniques. Subsequently, windowing can be applied to each component separately. Once the dense regions are defined as a region of interest, intensity windowing is applied to that area.

Contrast Limited Adaptive Histogram Equalization

Contrast Limited Adaptive Histogram Equalization (CLAHE) is a subtype of the class of algorithms known as Adaptive Histogram Equalization (AHE). Through AHE, the image's histogram is reset for smaller subsets of pixels producing locally calculated histograms. These local histograms are then equalized or remapped from the often-narrow range of intensity values indicative of a central pixel and its closest neighbors to the full range of intensity values available in the display. CLAHE sets a maximum limit to the contrast that will be displayed in each local histogram. CLAHE parameter settings (clip and region size) must be decided in advance of their application to the images. For the IDMDG preference study, a preliminary study was performed to attempt to determine the best specific values for clip and region size (7). Subsequently, MIW is applied to the image to adjust the contrast to levels to more closely resemble standard screen-film mammography. Of course, MIW can be replaced by other automated IW algorithms for this last step as well.

MUSICA

MUSICA (Agfa Division of Bayer Corporation, Ridgefield Park, NJ) is a multiscale wavelet-based processing algorithm that enhances the visibility of low-contrast structures. MUSICA processing also has parameters that must be adjusted based on preliminary decisions about image quality and diagnostic accuracy. For the IDMDG preference study, MUSICA itself was set at a maximum parameter value with the other MUSICA parameters set to 0.

Unsharp Masking

Unsharp masking (UM) (8,9) creates a low-pass filtered version of the original image and this new image subsequently subtracted from the original image. The resulting high-pass image is then added to the original image. This produces the final image with accentuated edges. Manual intensity windowing (or an automated IW algorithm) can then be applied to the image to adjust the contrast to levels more closely resembling standard screen-film mammography.

Peripheral Equalization

Peripheral Equalization (PE) enhances the periphery of the breast, an area that is not well seen on screen-film because the number of photons available to make an image puts the system into the shoulder of the H and D curve (See Fig. 2-4). This is because of the variations of thickness in the breast tissue under compression with the thinnest portions of the breast located at the periphery. With PE, a significantly less-detailed version of the mammogram is used to approximate breast thickness. Thresholding is then applied to the resulting image and extended circumferentially a bit to determine exactly where the breast skin line is located. Ideally, this algorithm should not affect the contrast available for viewing the interior, denser regions of the breast. After PE is applied, MIW (or an automated IW algorithm) can be applied to adjust the resulting image contrast to more closely resemble a screen-film mammogram (10).

Trex-Processing

Trex-processing was developed by Trex for use with the Trex digital mammography acquisition system. This method utilizes a form of histogram-based unsharp masking. It is a proprietary algorithm with the exact details held confidential by the company, so that no further information about it is available.

THE EFFECTS OF IMAGE PROCESSING ON LESION CHARACTERIZATION AND LESION DETECTION

For each machine included in the IDMDG preference study, there was a statistically significant relationship between lesion type and image processing algorithm preference for lesion characterization. That is, for all machines, radiologists preferred different algorithms for the characterization of masses and for the characterization of calcifications. Given the study design, one would expect that these results would apply to other digital mammography units developed in the future as well.

Fischer Lesion Characterization and Detection

For the Fischer images with masses (including masses with calcifications) undergoing characterization, all printed digital mammograms were preferred to the screen-film mammograms for all eight processing algorithms, with Musica, Trex processing, PE, UM and CLAHE significantly preferred. For the diagnostic evaluation of calcifications, three of the eight printed digital mammograms, Trex processing, HIW, and MMIW, were rated as slightly better or equivalent to the screen-film mammograms but these differences were not statistically significant. The screen-film images were significantly favored over the MIW and PE processed digital mammograms (11).

For the detection of both masses and calcifications in the Fischer images, only Trex processed-digital radiographs were preferred to screen-film mammograms, although they were not strongly preferred. The screen-film image was strongly preferred over the MMIW-processed images for both mass and calcification detection. The screen-film image was also strongly preferred over MIW, PE and UM for the detection of calcifications.

GE Lesion Characterization and Detection

For the mass diagnostic task with the GE images, the UM processed digital image was slightly but not statistically significantly preferred to the screen-film image. The screen-film mammogram was statistically significantly preferred over the Trex processed images. For the calcifications diagnostic task with the GE images, the MIW, HIW, UM, MMIW processed images were all slightly preferred to the screen-film mammograms. However, no digital processing algorithm was statistically significantly preferred. The screen-film mammogram was statistically significantly preferred over the PE processed images.

For the detection of both masses and calcifications in the GE images, the screen-film mammograms were preferred to the printed digital radiographs for all processing algorithms. These preferences were all quite strong, except for Musica and HIW for masses, and Musica and MIW for calcifications.

Trex Lesion Characterization and Detection

For the mass diagnostic task and the Trex images, all processed digital images except MMIW were preferred to the film-screen mammogram, with the Trex and HIW images statistically significantly preferred. The film-screen mammogram was slightly, but not statistically significantly preferred to the MMIW image. For the diagnostic evaluation of calcifications in the Trex images, the screen-film radiograph was statistically significantly preferred over all eight processed digital images. These results were statistically significant for all eight algorithms.

The Trex-processed digital radiograph for the detection of masses was the only processing method preferred to the screen-film mammogram, but it was not strongly preferred. The screen-film mammogram was preferred to all other processed digital images for the detection of masses. The screen-film mammogram was strongly preferred to all eight processed digital images for the detection of calcifications.

Other Machine Types

Since the IDMDG study did not include other machine types, it is unknown which of these image processing algorithms can improve lesion characterization or lesion detection for those machines. It is important to realize that the results for the Trex system may not apply to the Hologic system because the physics of image acquisition for the two systems are fundamentally different, even though the same company produces the two systems.

For examples of the appearance of the different image processing algorithms for different lesion types (see Figs. 7-1 to 7-4).

SUMMARY

As can be seen from these results, the radiologists preferred different processing methods for the diagnosis of masses than for the diagnosis of calcifications, and the preferred method varied by machine type. In addition, processing methods preferred for the purpose of screening differed from those chosen for lesion characterization or diagnosis, and the manufacturer's preselected algorithms (the default algorithms provided with the softcopy display system provided by that company) were not always the best ones for the tasks to be performed in the judgment of breast imaging experts.

The results of this study suggest that multiple presentations should be utilized for optimal digital mammography interpretation. Thus, at least three different presentations may be desirable for the same case (a screening presentation, a presentation to evaluate calcifications, and a presentation to evaluate masses) (1). As was mentioned in Chapter 6, this suggests that the ideal method of image presentation should be a softcopy system, perhaps with a computer aided diagnosis system activated so as to provide the optimal image processing locally applied to the regions where lesions are detected by the computer. In such a manner, radiologists would be able to view the images ideally without having to manipulate them too much, saving valuable interpretation time, and assuring that the ideal presentation format was used for every section of each case.

Given these results and those of others (7–9), the diagnostic accuracy of digital mammography will depend not only on the acquisition device itself, but also on the processing method utilized for image display. Further, if poor choices are made, diagnostic accuracy might be worse than for screen-film mammography. It is extremely important for the success of this new technology for radiologists and technologists to determine what image processing methods would be appropriate both for screening and the diagnostic evaluation of calcifications and masses.

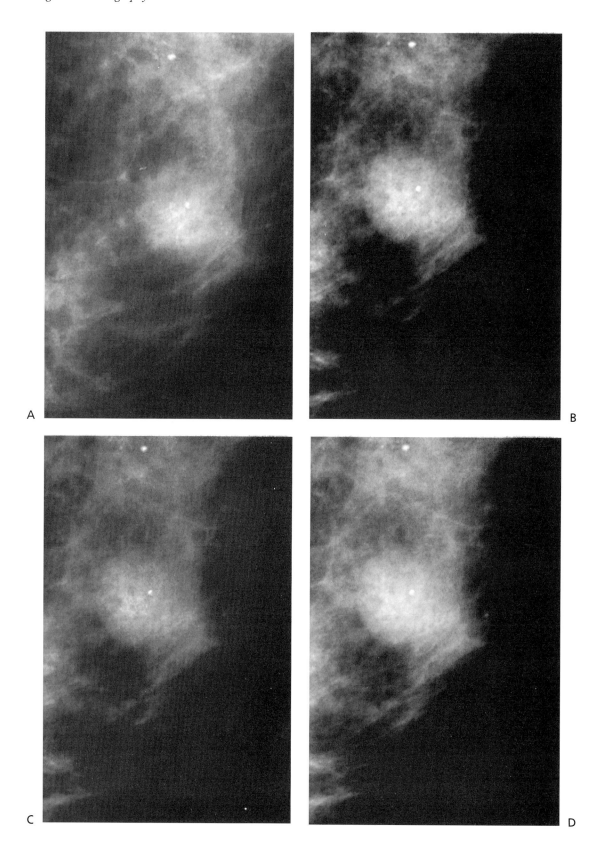

A

B

C

D

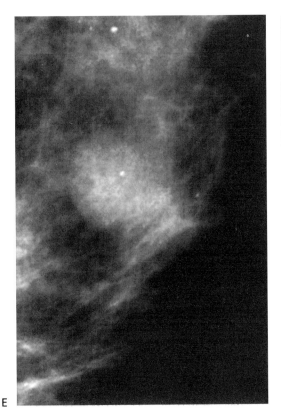

E

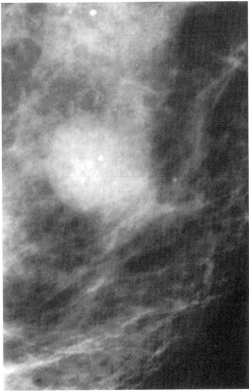

F

G

FIGURE 7-1. **(A)** A screen-film mammogram with a mass with indistinct and obscured borders. The radiologists preferred all versions of the Fischer digital mammogram to the screen-film image for this patient. The same mass displayed in the MMIW-processed digital mammogram is much more conspicuous **(B).** However, note the loss of conspicuity of the peripheral fat in this image. This is an undesirable feature for the screening task, but is irrelevant to the characterization task. CLAHE **(C),** MIW **(D),** and UM **(E)** processed images all show improved conspicuity of the mass, but loss of detail in the periphery of the breast. While the mass borders are less clear in the PE processed image **(F),** the periphery of the breast is more obvious with PE than in the screen-film examination, displaying an advantage of this algorithm. HIW **(G),** was also preferred by the radiologists to the screen-film mammogram for this case. (Reproduced with permission from Pisano ED, Cole EB, Hemminger BM, et al. Image processing algorithms for digital mammography: A pictorial essay. RadioGraphics 2000;20: 1479–1491.)

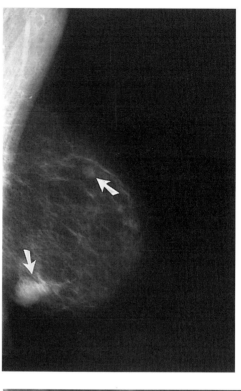
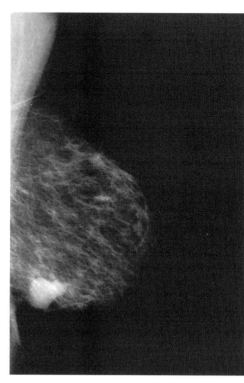

A, B

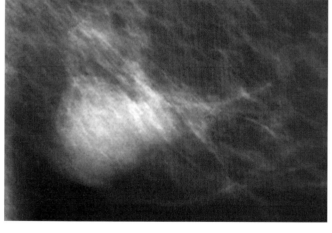

C

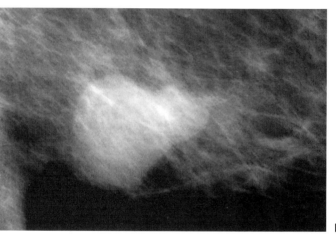

D

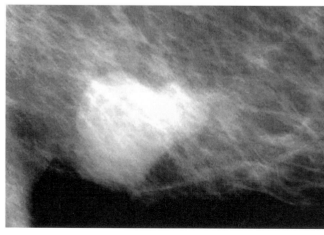

E

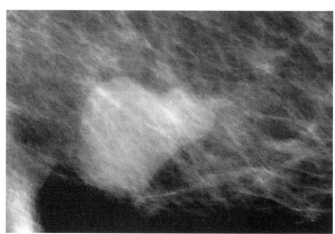

F

FIGURE 7-2. (A and C) display a screen-film mammogram with two masses (arrows), both pathologically proven infiltrating ductal carcinomas with associated ductal carcinoma in situ, with a photographic close-up of the larger lesion shown in **(C-F).** The GE digital mammogram, displayed with MMIW **(D)** MIW **(E),** and UM **(F),** were all considered better than the screen-film examination. The MIW image makes some portions of the mass excessively light, but its border visibility is maintained. The MMIW processed image improves mass conspicuity, but there is loss of fatty tissue surrounding the lesion that was not so severe that the periphery of the breast could not still be seen. This is especially noticeable when viewing the entire breast **(B)**. (Reproduced with permission from Pisano ED, Cole EB, Hemminger BM, et al. Image processing algorithms for digital mammography: A pictorial essay. RadioGraphics 2000; 20:1479–1491. Film and digital mammogram provided by Daniel Kopans of Massachusetts General Hospital.)

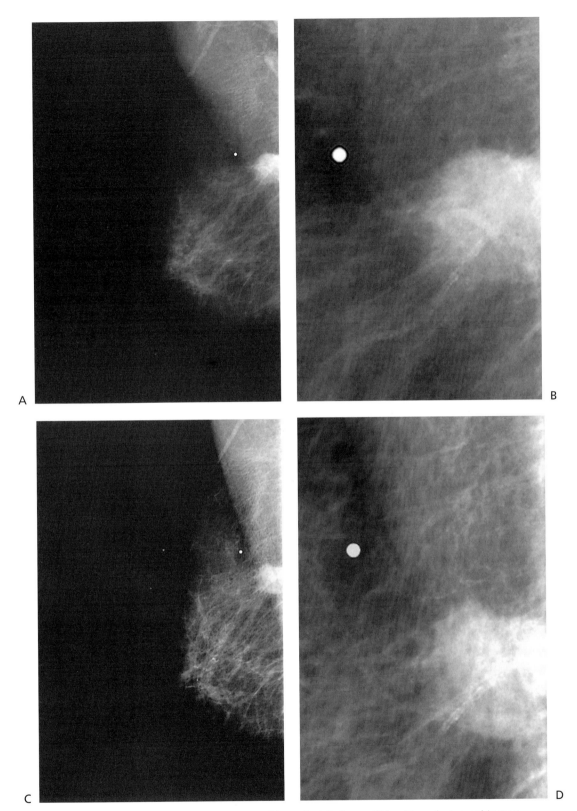

A

B

C

D

FIGURE 7-3. A screen-film mammogram with a spiculated mass **(A)**, with a photographic magnification of the lesion shown in **(B)**. The only Fischer digital processed image which was judged superior to the screen-film for viewing this mass was the UM image **(C)**. The center of the mass appears light but the spiculations are more clearly defined, especially in this photographic magnification of the digital and screen-film mammograms **(B,D)**. Slight differences in positioning and compression may contribute some of this apparent improvement. (Reproduced with permission from Pisano ED, Cole EB, Hemminger BM, et al. Image processing algorithms for digital mammography: A pictorial essay. RadioGraphics 2000;20:1479–1491.)

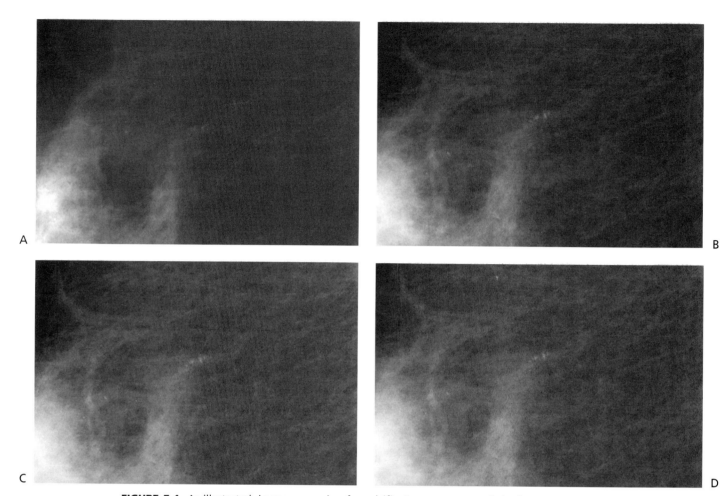

FIGURE 7-4. As illustrated, image processing for calcifications may cause their disappearance. **(A)** A screen-film mammogram containing a cluster of benign calcifications in a mostly fatty region. Every processed version of this Trex digital mammogram (provided by Laurie Fajardo and the University of Virginia) was deemed superior to the film-screen image for the characterization of these calcifications, as illustrated in **(A)** through **(H)**. The CLAHE processed image **(B)** was judged best for this task. All other processed algorithms, namely, MMIW **(C)**, HIW **(D)**, MIW **(E)**, Trex **(F)**, PE **(G)** and UM **(H)**, also provided good visualization of these calcifications. PE and UM processed images were believed to be too dark for this case, causing the calcifications to be visible but less conspicuous. (Reproduced with permission from Pisano ED, Cole EB, Hemminger BM, et al. Image processing algorithms for digital mammography: A pictorial essay. RadioGraphics 2000;20:1479–1491.)

Unfortunately, the manufacturers of digital mammography equipment have treated image processing as a "black box," that is, proprietary, not for public scrutiny. They do not provide a lot of information to the readers of the studies regarding what they have done to the images to make them more attractive. Of course, aesthetics should not be the only criterion driving decisions regarding mammography display. It is important that decisions regarding image processing be driven by improvements in diagnostic accuracy.

As has been demonstrated by the preference study cited here, the sorts of studies that should be performed do not have to be large and expensive, with huge numbers of abnormal mammograms included to decide basic issues regarding how images should be displayed to reveal the maximum amount of useful information to sophisticated readers. The Susan G. Komen Foundation has recently funded another study of image processing algorithms to help determine whether the companies have selected the appropriate algorithms for the display of their images or whether different

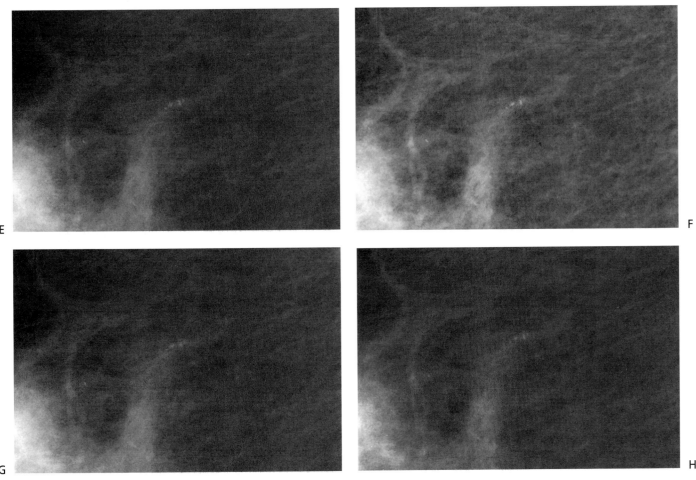

E

F

G

H

FIGURE 7-4. *continued.*

types of processing would be useful to improve the diagnostic accuracy achievable through digital mammography.

REFERENCES

1. Pisano ED, Cole EB, Major S, et al. Radiologists' preferences for digital mammographic display. Radiology 2000;216(3): 820–830.
2. Puff DT, Cromartie R, Pisano ED. Evaluation and optimization of contrast enhancement methods for medical images. Proc SPIE Visualization Biom Comput Conf 1992;1808:336–346.
3. Puff DT, Pisano ED, Muller KE, et al. A method for determination of optimal image enhancement for the detection of mammographic abnormalities. J Dig Imaging 1994;7: 161–171.
4. Pisano ED, Chandramouli J, Hemminger BM, et al. Does intensity windowing improve the detection of simulated calcifications in dense mammograms? J Dig Imaging 1007;10(2): 79–84.
5. Pisano ED, Chandramouli J, Hemminger BM, et al. The effect of intensity windowing as an image processing tool in the detection of simulated masses embedded in digitized mammograms. J Dig Imaging 1997;10(4):174–182.
6. Pisano ED, Zong S, Hemminger BM, et al. Contrast limited adaptive histogram equalization image processing to improve the detection of simulated spiculations in dense mammograms. J Dig Imaging 1998B;11(4):193–200.
7. Oestmann JW, Kopans D, Hall DA, et al. A comparison of digitized storage phosphors and conventional mammography in the detection of malignant microcalcifications. Invest Radiol 1988; 23:725–728.
8. Cowen AR, Brettle DS, Coleman NJ, et al. A preliminary investigation of the imaging performance of photostimulable phosphor computed radiography using a new design of mammographic quality control test object. Br J Radiol 1992;65: 528–535.
9. Higashida Y, Morida N, Morita K, et al. Detection of subtle microcalcifications: Comparison of computed radiography and screen-film mammography. Radiology 1992;183: 483–486.
10. Byng JW, Critten JP, Yaffe MJ. Thickness equalization processing for mammographic images. Radiology 1997;203:564–568.
11. Puff D, Pisano E, Johnston E, et al. The effects of CLAHE on simulated mammographic object detection. J Dig Imaging 1994; 7(4):161–17.

8

IMAGE DISPLAY: SOFTCOPY AND PRINTED FILM BASICS OF DIGITAL MAMMOGRAPHY DISPLAY

ETTA D. PISANO

As has been detailed in previous chapters, different digital mammography systems acquire mammograms at different levels of spatial and contrast resolution. Spatial resolution ranges from 41 μ per pixel for the Trex/Lorad system to 100 μ per pixel for the General Electric (GE) system. Contrast resolution ranges from 10 bits per pixel for the Fuji Computed Radiography system to 14 bits per pixel for the GE and Trex/Lorad systems.

Bit depth is defined as a power of 2. A system with a bit depth of 12 provides 2^{12} (or 4,096) gray levels in every pixel. The system translates the photons captured by its detector into 4,096 possible gray levels, from the blackest black to the whitest white with 4,094 shades in between.

However, the radiologist reader needs to know more than how the image is acquired to understand the limitations of the information available in evaluating a digital image. The method used for image display further defines the performance of the system, and the information that is available to the reader. Of course, the display medium is limited in both size and bit depth.

The issue of size will be addressed first. The assumption is that a mammogram is one of two standard sizes, 18×24 cm or 24×30 cm, as produced by the Fuji CR system. That system consists of digital detectors that are used in place of mammography cassettes with traditional film mammography tubes. The image acquired can be printed to films of the same size as the detector. If this happens, the pixels are all printed without any loss of size when compared to the original image at acquisition. The reader can employ a magnifying glass to see the smallest objects visible in the image, including those confined to just a few pixels or less.

Of course, the image could be printed on film of a larger size than the detector that was used at the time of image acquisition. If that were done, each pixel would take up more space on the film in absolute area than the original object took up within the breast and at the detector at acquisition. This would make each pixel larger to the reader reviewing the image. It is possible that because of this mag-

nification, the user will not need a magnifying lens to see the smallest objects in the image. Note that there is no more information available to the reader with this sort of enlargement technique. The smallest objects visible in the image are merely made more obvious.

Similarly, the image could be printed on film of a size smaller than the detector. This will shrink the image, and the pixels will take up less absolute area than they did at the time of image acquisition. This will have no real advantage to the reader, of course, because the smallest size objects in the image (i.e., those that can be seen by most readers only with a magnifying glass) will be even smaller, making some of the smallest objects imperceptible to most readers.

A similar discussion is applicable to display of the images using softcopy systems. Monitors can provide display of the images at exactly the same size as the original acquisition, at a smaller size, or at a larger size. The only way one can be sure of seeing all the image detail visible at acquisition is to view the image at the same size at which it was acquired. One can use magnifying lenses, either virtual or real, to make the images relatively bigger, but that does not add detail to the images. It does improve the relative visibility of what is indeed in the image, of course.

So, in viewing any digital image on a monitor, it is important to know how the image is being seen relative to its full spatial resolution Currently, only cathode ray tube (CRT) monitor technology is available for the softcopy display of digital mammograms. These typically provide 2,048 × 2,560 pixels displayed over monitor sizes of 30 × 40 cm. While some mammograms can be displayed at full resolution in their entirety on typical workstation monitors (e.g., those acquired on the GE system at 100 μ spatial resolution), the Fischer mammograms, for example, contain 3,072 × 4,800 pixels. This means that the monitors can only display part of the mammogram at full resolution at any one time. Radiologists need to see both the overview of the images compared to the opposite breast, old films for comparison (to look for asymmetries, masses, and gross changes), and fine detail only visible at full spatial resolution with magnification applied. Therefore, the softcopy systems must provide some sort of "roam and zoom" functionality, which means that the images must first be brought up at lower than full spatial resolution. Then the user must systematically navigate through the whole image at full spatial resolution, with or without further magnification. This is the only way users can be certain that they have viewed the whole image with the smallest detail visible for review.

Similarly, the contrast available in a digital image can be displayed on film or on a monitor. If the images are printed to film by a laser printer, this typically is done with 10 to 12 bits per pixel displayed. If the image at acquisition contained more than 12 bits, then the contrast in the image needs to be remapped to the number of bits available for display.

For example, for an image acquired at 14 bits with 16,384 gray levels assigned and now displayed with only 4,096 possible gray levels, the contrast scale must be compressed. Similar to the use of intensity windowing for computed tomography, the user must define how the image will look by choosing how the gray levels will be compressed for display. The simplest remapping involves just assigning every four gray levels in order from blackest to whitest to the corresponding gray level in the new compressed scale from blackest to whitest for an image displayed at 12 bits per pixel. Similarly, every 16 consecutive gray levels would be assigned to the corresponding gray levels in the compressed scale for an image displayed at 10 bits per pixel. For film display, that is the end of the story. There is no way to retrieve the additional contrast information from the raw digital data.

Similarly, monitors do not allow the full range of contrast resolution to be displayed at any one time. The typical CRT monitor display has a bit depth of eight. This means it displays only 2^8, or 256, gray levels at any one time. The user (or manufacturer) can set up the contrast in the image to be displayed in any way that is desired. Again, that might involve compressing the gray scale from the original 16,384 gray levels (for a 14-bit image) to the 256 available on the 8-bit monitor by assigning 2^6 or 64 gray levels in the original image to every gray level displayed on the monitor.

However, that is not the end of the story with softcopy display. Given the dynamic nature of these systems, the user has the flexibility to reset the gray level across the entire gray scale. Users, if they choose, can systematically search through the entire range of gray values that could be assigned to the image. This might be especially needed for patients with dense breasts where there are subtle differences in contrast across the densest parts of the breast.

Of course, accessing the additional information in the image by roaming and zooming and changing the gray levels takes the reader time. Ideally, such tools should be set up so that they are as simple to use as possible, without requiring too much active attention from the reader. Display tools that distract radiologists while they are interpreting images can actually harm diagnostic accuracy. Thus, the emphasis by the Food and Drug Administration (FDA) on the separate approval process for softcopy display systems. The tools must be carefully designed not only to allow the proper display of the images, but also to allow the user to manipulate the images to see all available image detail without undue distraction.

Another big difference between softcopy display systems and film display on a monitor is the brightness, or the luminance, available in the images. Viewbox luminance is measured in candelas per m^2, also known as nits. A nit is the amount of light either reflected or emitted by a surface. The American College of Radiology (ACR) and the United States Agency for Health Care Policy and Research recommend that viewbox luminance levels for mammography be at least 3,000 nits, or 878 fL (1,2). In contrast, the luminance levels for high brightness monitors are approximately 514 nits, or 150 fL.

Does this difference in luminance really affect diagnostic accuracy? Two studies have demonstrated that mammography feature detection performance does not decrease when softcopy display luminance ranges are used instead of mammography lightbox ranges (3,4). However, larger scale performance studies evaluating the effect of display characteristics on the detection and diagnosis of breast cancer are required to assure patients and physicians that film and softcopy display are equivalent. The preliminary data on the diagnostic accuracy of film versus softcopy display with CRT monitors will be presented in the next section.

ADDITIONAL INFORMATION ON PRINTING TO FILM

Laser printers for digital mammography are available from several vendors. They support spatial resolutions comparable to screen-film mammography (up to 4,800 × 6,400 pixel matrix size) and with the reproduced size capable of matching the acquisition resolutions of current scanners (down to 41 μ pixel size). The gray scale range is roughly similar to that of mammography film, with laser-printed films achieving maximum optical density (OD) of 3.5 to 4.0, while mammography films can achieve maximum ODs slightly greater than 4.0. Laser-printed films generally are not subject to the same level of processor variability or processor artifacts that are present with single-emulsion screen-film mammograms. Furthermore, laser-printed films allow radiologists to use the same reading protocols as they are currently using in interpreting screen-film images. Films can be hung on a multipanel viewer with standardized layout, and a "hot light" and magnifying lens can be easily utilized. This takes advantage of the significant training and familiarity that radiologists have in interpreting screen-film mammograms.

The disadvantages of using laser-printed film are cost and the availability of only on presentation format per sheet of film. The costs include the time expended for printing and development, as well as the personnel and supplies needed for these tasks. Furthermore, if more than one processed version is needed to extract the maximum amount of information from a mammogram, more than one version should be printed. This is of course quite impractical, especially in a screening setting where speed and efficiency are essential to the goal of cost containment. An additional disadvantage of film display is the loss of dynamic range inherent in displaying a 12- to 14-bit image at 8 bits. As detailed above, printed film generally can display a wider range of the contrast inherent in the image, often up to 12 bits.

CLINICAL STUDIES OF SOFTCOPY DISPLAY

In fact, several early clinical studies of digital mammography that compare softcopy to printed film display have suggested that the use of softcopy may improve specificity by reducing false–positive examinations. This would presumably be achieved because of the flexible display of the examinations that is possible with softcopy display. This allows the user to manipulate the images to determine whether something is a composite density or a real lesion.

One large study compared the speed and accuracy of the interpretation of Fischer digital mammograms on softcopy versus those on film (5). The softcopy system used was developed at the University of North Carolina (UNC) and was similar to the one Fischer eventually developed for its commercial digital mammography system. The images were printed using the manufacturer's recommended algorithm. After training in digital mammography interpretation, 8 radiologists interpreted 63 digital mammograms, all with old studies for comparison. All studies were interpreted by all readers in softcopy and on printed film, with interpretations of the same cases at least one month apart. Cases included 6 biopsy-proven cancers and 13 biopsy-proven benign lesions, as well as 23 patients who underwent six-month follow-up for probably benign findings and 20 cases that were considered normal by virtue of one year of mammographic and clinical follow-up.

The results of this study showed that there was a tendency for interpretations on softcopy to be slightly faster than film interpretations, with mean reading times of 34 versus 40.5 seconds respectively. In contrast, the area under the receiver operator characteristic (ROC) curve (0.67 film, 0.65 softcopy) and sensitivity (0.71 film, 0.69 softcopy) were slightly better for film than softcopy, but specificity was slightly better for softcopy (0.563) than for film (0.528). However, none of these results was statistically significant, possibly because of the small sample size in the study (5).

In addition, as described in Chapter 4, the large screening trial performed by Lewin and his colleagues also showed fewer call backs and a lower biopsy rate when digital softcopy interpretations were compared with screen-film interpretations for the same patients (6). These investigators hypothesized that this may have been the result of the improved flexibility of image display available with the softcopy system that was used. By manipulating image data, radiologists might be able to figure out whether "lesions" are real or the result of overlapping shadows or other artifacts, without having the patients undergo additional imaging.

Of course, it is also possible that this improvement in specificity could be the result of reduced sensitivity, that is, if the digital detector finds fewer clustered calcifications and masses than film mammography, since most detected lesions are benign, the specificity would be improved if fewer lesions were found overall. This cause for increased specificity for calcifications was tested in a recent study by the International Digital Mammography Development Group, which was reported at the Radiologic Society of North America 2002 meeting (7). In that study, the digital and screen-film mammograms of 130 patients with calcifications were evaluated by eight radiologists. The readers were asked to rate the probability of malignancy just for the clusters of calcifications with the images cropped on the softcopy system or film just to include the regions of interest. The monitor system provided roam and zoom and intensity windowing capability for the readers, and readers could use magnifying lenses with both systems. The digital system showed a nonsignificant tendency toward higher specificity (83.3% vs. 80.3%). While the results were nonsignificant and must be confirmed through larger studies in a more realistic clinical situation, they support the trend in the literature toward improved specificity when softcopy systems are used.

Finally, Sickles has demonstrated that remote interpretation of digital mammograms by a radiologist using a softcopy system across town can be done statistically significantly faster than the interpretation of film mammograms with the radiologist reading them in the same facility. The gain in time was attributed to the fact that the digital mammograms did not have to undergo processing, as film mammograms do. They were available for interpretation faster, even across town, because they could be interpreted within a few seconds (rather than a few minutes) of their acquisition (8).

FUTURE TRENDS IN DISPLAY OF DIGITAL MAMMOGRAMS

Other technologies, such as liquid crystal display, field emission display, and organic light emitting diode displays, should become available for the softcopy display of mammograms in the next few years (9). The effects on diagnostic accuracy of these new monitor systems are not known yet, of course, but it seems likely that these technologies will have only small incremental benefit compared to the current CRT technology.

More promising would be the availability of an "intelligent workstation" (10), as was described in Chapter 6. Such a viewing system is not yet commercially available but could become so in the next few years. Specifically, it would provide very fast computer-aided diagnosis (CAD) with immediate image processing and annotation of the regions of interest (10). For example, if the CAD system suggested the presence of a cluster of calcifications, the images could be viewed with the region that probably contained the lesion circled on the image with the image processing algorithm that is best for detecting calcifications (as determined by systematic reader studies like the one described in Chapter 7) automatically applied to that region of interest. If the reader then zoomed in on the area, the machine could automatically switch from the best algorithm for detection to the best algorithm for characterization of calcifications. If designed properly, with rigorous attention to ergonomic issues so that the interface does not distract the user, such workstations could seamlessly and automatically provide viewing conditions that are appropriate for the goals of the reader and the circumstances of the patient (i.e., whether she has a probably normal or probably abnormal digital mammogram). That is, different tools might be provided for screening and diagnosis and different display parameters might be set for mammograms with lesions detected versus those without lesions. While these sorts of tools are not available at present, they are can be developed in the near future and, in my judgment, they are very likely to positively affect the diagnostic accuracy of digital mammography.

REFERENCES

1. American College of Radiology (ACR) Committee on Quality Assurance in Mammography. Mammography Quality Control. Reston, VA: ACR, 1999;68–70,142,185–196,208–209,287–294.
2. Bassett LW, Hendrick RE, Bassford TL, et al. Quality Determinants of Mammography: Clinical Practice Guideline No. 13. Rockville, MD: Agency for Health Care Policy and Research. Public Health Service, U.S. Department of Health and Human Services. 1994:65 (publication no. 95-0632).
3. Roehrig H, Krupinski E. Image Quality of CRT displays and the effect of brightness of diagnosis of mammograms. J Digit Imaging 1998;11(3 Suppl 1):87–188.
4. Hemminger BM, Sthapit S, Pisano ED. Demonstration of a softcopy display system for digital mammography (abstract). Radiology 1998;213:583.
5. Pisano ED, Cole EB, Kistner EO, et al. Digital mammography interpretation: Comparison of the speed and accuracy of softcopy versus printed film display. Radiology 2001;223:483–488.
6. Lewin JM, D'Orsi CJ, Hendrick RE, et al. Clinical comparison of full field digital mammography and screen-film mammography for detection of breast cancer. AJR 2002;179:671–677.
7. Kim HH, Pisano ED, Cole EB, et al. Comparison of specificity for calcifications in digital mammograms using softcopy versus film (abstract). Radiology 2002;225(P)(Suppl):416.
8. Sickles EA. Computer-aided diagnosis and telemammography: Clinical perspective. In: Haus AG, Yaffe MJ, eds. Physical Aspects of Breast Imaging: Current and Future Considerations. RSNA Publications, Chicago, Il. 1999:283–285.
9. Shtern F, Winfield D (eds). Report of the working group on digital mammography: Digital displays and workstation design. Acad Radiol 1999;6:S197–S218.
10. Doi K, Giger ML, Nishikawa RM, et al. Computer-aided diagnosis of breast cancer on mammograms. Breast Cancer 1997;4:228–233.

9

PACS ISSUES

FRED M. BEHLEN

Some form of Picture Archiving and Communications System (PACS) is generally required to make a digital mammography system economically viable. The diagnostic benefits of digital mammography are attended by substantial expenditures for equipment and its maintenance. These costs need to be offset by cost savings and higher productivity if digital mammography is to be adopted in breast imaging departments already under economic pressure.

Successful and efficient mammography reporting must bring together the current and prior images, prior reports, orders and other clinical information, and the reporting or dictation systems used to create the reports. While DICOM standards allow the connection of image acquisition units, displays, archives and reporting systems from different vendors, the practical integration of these devices usually hinges on a balance of technical and business factors. A key decision in many settings will be whether to acquire a "Mammography PACS," usually bundled with the digital mammography system, or to use a departmental PACS resource. This chapter seeks to inform the reader in the issues of such a choice, beginning with a basic review of systems.

BASICS OF PICTURE ARCHIVING AND COMMUNICATIONS SYSTEM

Figure 9-1 illustrates schematically the information flows of diagnostic imaging and is applicable to either filmless or hardcopy practice. Images are acquired and sent to the image display, along with images of prior examinations retrieved from storage. Current images are also stored for future use as "priors," either directly or, as in the case of hardcopy practice, after viewing. The radiologist reviews the images, together with the referring physician's order, prior reports, and other clinical data, and then creates the report sent to the referring physician and inserted in the medical record.

A PACS serves the image-handling aspects of this process. There are five principal functions of a PACS:

1. Image Acquisition: Interfacing with the digital imaging equipment and receiving the digital image data.
2. Image Storage: Securely storing the image data, which may total may thousands of gigabytes.
3. Image Communication: Rapidly communicating image data over computer networks.
4. Image Display: Formatting and displaying images on workstation screens sufficient for primary diagnosis or for other clinical tasks.
5. Image Management: Properly identifying and indexing the data in terms of its clinical context.

These functional areas correspond to five specialized core competencies that have traditionally distinguished PACS manufacturers, but many of these functions are now served by mass-market technologies. Conventional desktop personal computers are available with 100-gigabyte disk drives and 100 megabit-per-second network adapters. Displaying pictures on computer screens is routine, and although medical imaging displays still have important performance advantages in brightness and resolution, that gap is being closed by general-market liquid crystal display (LCD) devices. Thus, the capability to efficiently manage and present image data is becoming the core value added by PACS vendors.

Figure 9-2 depicts the basic elements of a digital breast imaging facility's imaging and information systems. Images acquired by the digital mammography unit are initially displayed in an acquisition workstation that often serves as the operator's console as well. Images may be reviewed for proper positioning by the technologist and are then sent over the computer network to the archive. Some acquisition workstations can also automatically send the images directly to the diagnostic workstation. The figure also shows a laser film printer, still a common fixture as some hardcopy is occasionally needed even in "filmless" practices.

The core component of what is usually called a PACS is the PACS Archive, comprising an image manager and an image archive, as shown in Figure 9-2. The Image Archive provides short-term image storage on magnetic disks, and generally provides for long-term archival storage on removable media, such as optical disks or high-density magnetic

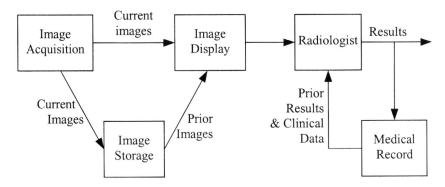

FIGURE 9-1. Information Flows in Diagnostic Imaging

tape cartridges. Robotic libraries are often used to automate the retrieval of off-line media, and such robotically retrievable media are usually called "near-line." The image manager is the "brains" of the PACS, directing automated flows of images and performing administrative and management functions. Separate computers may perform image manager and image archive functions, but from both a procurement and an operational standpoint, they are commonly treated as a unit. The PACS archive sends prior images to the diagnostic workstation, which also receives the current images, either directly from the acquisition workstation or relayed from the archive. The figure also shows an ultrasound scanner, as a reminder that a digital mammography PACS must often integrate with other breast imaging devices as well.

A final element in Figure 9-2, labeled "Information System(s)," represents a collection of functions sometimes served by a dedicated mammography reporting system, but often distributed among several departmental and enterprise systems as follows:

- Scheduling.
- Registration.
- Workflow management.
- Reporting/dictation.
- Follow-up.
- Quality assurance.
- Billing.

The efficiency that a digital mammography operation must achieve depends on the smooth integration of the information system functions with image acquisition, storage, and display, a fact that a block diagram cannot adequately communicate. We will address these integration issues more fully, after first placing the data storage requirement in appropriate perspective.

Storage Requirements

Many people speak of the mammoth data sets produced by digital mammography examinations, but such data sets still

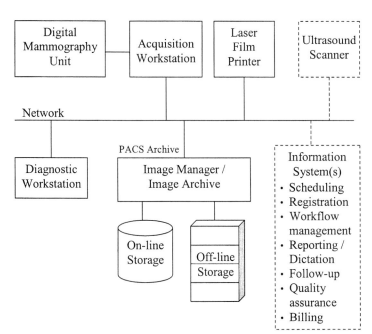

FIGURE 9-2. Information System in a Breast Imaging Facility

represent only a fraction of the amount of data that can be stored on a recordable CD costing US $0.30. The size of mammography data sets is also no problem for today's local area networks. A 40-MB mammogram can be transferred between commodity personal computers in fewer than seven seconds. And, just as the capacity of inexpensive computing hardware has increased to match the needs of digital mammography, so the space demands of other imaging modalities have also grown to a level comparable to that of mammography. Current multiplane helical CT scanners routinely produce 50 megabyte data sets from a single breath-hold.

It is difficult to generalize the space requirements for mammography PACS, because at this time, the spatial resolution of commercial digital mammography systems vary widely, from as little as 10 MB per image to 50 MB per image, or from 16 MB to 80 MB per four-view screening examination, after applying lossless data compression at 2.5:1. At the low-resolution end of this range, these image files are little larger than those of chest x-rays, at 4 MB per image using the same lossless compression ratio. In a good-sized hospital performing 180,000 radiology procedures per year, of which 10,000 are screening mammograms, the mammography storage would be on the order of 5% to 25% (depending on image size) of the storage capacity of the departmental PACS. Thus, the mammography data, while a significant addition to departmental storage load, could feasibly be accommodated by scaling of a departmental PACS.

At the other end of the complexity spectrum would be shelf management of digital mammograms stored on CD-R media. At 80 MB per exam after lossless compression, a standard 650 MB CD-R disk could store eight exams, resulting in a media cost (including jewel case) on the order of US $0.05 per exam (10 cents if a duplicate copy is made for off-site safe storage). The 10,000 exams would fill 1,250 CDs occupying 20 linear feet of shelf space in slim jewel cases, one two-foot-wide cabinet per year of storage. Placing images on 4.7 GB DVD-R media reduces the shelf space to 175 disks requiring less than three linear feet of

shelf space per year, at comparable media cost. The practicality of such a simple solution depends on the practice setting. It may work well in a dedicated imaging center, but may prove too difficult to manage in an academic medical center.

The space requirements of digital mammography are large, to be sure, but the point of the foregoing discussion is that their size is no longer qualitatively different from that of other imaging systems, and the special requirements of mammography PACS are as much practical and administrative as they are technical. Whether one does manual shelf-storage management, or incremental scaling of a departmental PACS, or any hybrid configuration in between, is a management decision rather than a technical one.

Mechanisms of Image Transmission

The mechanisms and formats of image transmission for digital mammography are one of the areas in which clear and well-accepted standards adequately serve the application needs. This is, in part, because the DICOM standard was already well developed and widely supported when digital mammography came on the scene, and the developers of the digital mammography image object benefited from past DICOM experience, with few constraints imposed by an installed base of prior versions.

DICOM mammography images are labeled with the modality code "MG" and are a specialization of the digital x-ray image object "DX." The DX image object was introduced in 1999 to more accurately support the needs of direct digital image capture devices. The digital mammography object is a specialization of the DX object, which requires that laterality and projection be present. It also provides useful optional fields for specifying the presence of implants and indicating partial views for large breasts. Projection geometry, position angles, and compression thickness may also be specified in the image object. View designations supported in the DICOM standard are shown in Table 9-1.

TABLE 9-1. DICOM VIEW AND VIEW MODIFIER DESIGNATIONS IN THE MAMMOGRAPHY (MG) IMAGE INFORMATION OBJECT

View	View Modifier	Applies only when view is:
Medio-lateral	Cleavage	CC
Medio-lateral oblique	Axillary tail	MLO
Latero-medial	Rolled lateral	Any
Latero-medial oblique	Rolled medial	Any
Cranio-caudal	Implant displaced	Any
Caudo-cranial (from below)	Magnification	Any
Superolateral to inferomedial oblique	Spot compression	Any
Exaggerated cranio-caudal	Tangential	Any
Cranio-caudal exaggerated laterally		
Cranio-caudal exaggerated medially		

Security Issues

Whenever identifiable patient information is handled on computer networks, heightened concern for privacy and security is appropriate. Although it is often noted that a person with a white lab coat and a confident demeanor can walk into many large medical facilities and see confidential information, such an intrusion requires far more personal risk than a hacker making an intrusion from afar. Heightened public concerns about security of personal information are now reflected in governmental regulations, such as those issued under the U.S. Health Information Portability and Accountability Act of 1996 (HIPAA). While the HIPAA privacy regulations have attracted much public discussion, the actual security measures they require differ little from the practices required by accreditation organizations such as Joint Commission Accreditations of Health Organizations (JCAHO). However, governmental regulations impose greater compliance assurance requirements and stiffer penalties for violators.

Because of the requirements for information access in emergency care, healthcare information security practices focus more on accountability than on restrictive security filters. That is, healthcare provider personnel are commonly given either broad access or the ability to override security filters, with the understanding that violation of access policies without valid emergency reasons will result in disciplinary action. The key requirements for this are the secure authentication of individual users, the maintenance of audit trails, and some kind of administrative procedures to monitor compliance.

The requirements of security regulations are that reasonable and appropriate measures are taken to ensure information security. No one measure is an absolute requirement. If a particular piece of equipment cannot feasibly be secured by user authentication, it may be necessary to improve physical security or monitoring of access to that equipment, but wholesale replacement or costly upgrade of imaging equipment is not what was envisioned by regulators.

The requirements for individual user log-ins may pose problems for shared equipment, such as viewing workstations and image acquisition systems. Some systems may base user authentication on log-in to the platform computer's operating system. On certain systems, when the user logs on, a large and complex suite of applications programs is brought up, requiring a minute or more. Such delays may be of no concern for a private office where the user logs in once in the morning but can be devastating in busy clinical environments with several users sharing access to a single machine. A different implementation approach by the system designer may leave the desktop and a set of applications programs running, but the applications programs would allow access only after log-in. Regulations also require automatic log-outs or screen-saver locks if the user walks away, as may be inferred from the absence of keyboard or mouse activity. This may cause significant inconvenience if the user is frequently called away.

The security issues discussed above are common to many PACS applications. The key conclusion is that although a number of technical and procedural approaches are available to meet security requirements and the various approaches are comparable in terms of the protection they offer to patients, approaches may differ dramatically in their impact on the workflow efficiency of a breast imaging facility. Those involved in system selection are well advised to involve both radiologists and technologists in a detailed walk-through of clinical procedures, including log-in, log-out, and interruptions.

Procurement Decisions

A major decision in procuring a digital mammography system will be between a "Mammography mini-PACS" or an addition to a departmental PACS. The advantages of using the departmental PACS for mammography are:

- Administrative simplicity. The department needs only a single set of skills, single set of training, single backup, single disaster recovery, and single system administration procedures.
- Enterprise distribution. Many departmental systems support image distribution to referring physicians through image Web servers or widely deployed client workstations. Physicians referring for mammography often do not need images, however.
- Scheduled workflow integration. If the mammography procedures are scheduled departmentally and the departmental PACS supports modality word lists for distribution of exam schedules and patient demographic data, the digital mammography suite may profitably use this resource to improve workflow.
- Reporting integration. It may be desirable (or institutionally mandated) to use the same dictation and reporting systems as other radiology reporting.

On the other hand, some considerations may make a dedicated Mammography PACS desirable:

- Procurement and installation simplicity. Mammography mini-PACS systems are often bundled with the imaging equipment, and managing the installation is considerably easier if connections to large departmental systems are forgone.
- Required retention times. Under U.S. law, mammography images must be stored indefinitely, whereas the general radiology images may be discarded after as few as five years (depending on state law and local standards). These differing retention times are handled most easily if the mammograms are stored on separate media.

- Business issues. Sometimes vendor pricing or packaging options significantly influence the economics of one approach or the other.

Thus, if one intends to add on to the department PACS, issues of concern are:

- Retention. Make sure the PACS is prepared to migrate the digital mammography data to successive systems, indefinitely, when the PACS is upgraded or replaced.
- Reporting system integration. If using a special mammography reporting system, consider how it will integrate with the PACS in the breast imaging center
- Suitability departmental prefetching and workflow tools. Make sure they will work for mammography.
- Potential clouding of responsibility between mammography and PACS vendors. Make sure both vendors agree to the acceptance criteria.

Conversely, procurement of a mammography mini-PACS involves the following concerns:

- Responsibility for system administration and backup procedures, which may remain in the breast imaging center with a mini-PACS.
- Disaster recovery procedures and maintenance of up-to-date off-site copies.
- Enterprise image distribution, depending on the needs of referring physicians for images.
- Integrating with the radiology information system for reporting, billing. and administrative functions.
- Interfacing with main PACS for retrieval of ultrasound images or other relevant images.
- Scheduled workflow integration. How will the scheduled exam lists and patient names get into the images? With-

out modality word lists, patient-identifying information must be keyboarded into imaging consoles, and errors may lead to incorrectly identified images.

Conclusion and Recommendations

Whether one undertakes to purchase a digital mammography system and integrate it with an existing PACS or to purchase a "turnkey" breast imaging system encompassing mammography and mammography mini-PACS, the best procurement strategy is not to avoid trying to become a technology expert. This is a challenge, rather than an excuse, for the clinical personnel involved in procurement decisions. An unfortunately common procurement approach is to state clinical requirements in broad terms and then distill them to detailed requirements at the technical level. The technical requirements then become embodied in the procurement contract. The problem is that compliance with detailed technical specifications will not guarantee the achievement of clinical goals. For example, it is better to specify how long it takes for the acquired image to get to the display than to specify its method of transmission or whether is routed through the archive unit. Therefore, a much better approach is to develop detailed clinical requirements. Work out in detail how each exam is performed, particularly all the steps that must be performed to complete the procedure, interpret it, and generate its report. Walk through these procedures with vendor personnel, clarifying and writing down how the system will work in your setting. Written notes from such walk-throughs will facilitate user training and serve as a valuable resource for resolving any misunderstandings with your suppliers.

10

ADVANCED APPLICATIONS OF DIGITAL MAMMOGRAPHY

MARTIN J. YAFFE

Digital mammography offers the potential for improved sensitivity and specificity for breast cancer imaging and for more efficient archiving and retrieval of mammograms. However, it may be the applications that can be built on the platform of digital mammography that make its clinical use most compelling and may ultimately justify the higher capital costs of this technology. One of these applications, computer aided diagnosis (CAD), was described in Chapter 6. Use of CAD with digital mammography eliminates the need for film digitization, and the higher quality data due to the extended dynamic range and higher signal-to-noise ratio (SNR) provided by the digital detector may result in improved accuracy of CAD algorithms. This chapter describes other applications that are under development. These include telemammography, tomosynthesis, contrast imaging, and measurement of mammographic density for risk assessment.

TELEMAMMOGRAPHY

In many communities, lack of access to an expert breast imager necessitates that mammograms are interpreted by general radiologists who may have neither the specialized training in mammography nor exposure to an adequate volume of work to keep their skills at the highest level. In other situations, radiologists may have to spend considerable unproductive time traveling to provide service to those communities. In yet another situation, in many large health care facilities, communication between the surgeon and the radiologist is inefficient because of the geographic separation of departments. Again, time is wasted by the need to have both individuals and images in the same location in order to carry out a consultation. Finally, because women may have moved or gone to a different facility since the previous mammography examination, and these facilities may be quite distant from one another, it is often difficult or impractical to obtain previous images for comparison to the current examination.

Digital mammography provides a perfect solution to these problems. As discussed in Chapter 9, a digital communication standard, DICOM, (1) has been developed to facilitate the transport of digital images between computers, and this standard has been refined to include a specialized module for digital mammography. Using digital images that conform to the DICOM mammography standard, it is convenient to transmit them from a digital mammography system to a remote diagnostic workstation for interpretation.

As shown in Table 10-1, digital mammograms are relatively large. Their size depends on the pixel size and the overall format of the receptor, but image size varies from approximately 9 MB for pixels that are 100 μ on a side to more than 45 MB for a 50 μ image. Considering that each examination usually produces at least four images and that a busy machine might handle 20–30 examinations per day, the amount of data that must be transmitted rapidly and accurately from a single mammography room is enormous—possibly 5 GB per day.

A telemammography system consists of one or more digital mammography units, linked by a network or communications line to one or more remote display workstations (Fig. 10-1). The success of a telemammography system also depends on several other key features. The system must contain appropriate software to facilitate image transmission. A database feature or Picture Archiving and Communications System PACS is necessary to allow tracking of

TABLE 10-1. SIZES IN MBYTES OF DIGITAL MAMMOGRAMS FOR VARIOUS PIXEL SIZES AND FORMATS

Image dimensions (cm)	Pixel size (μm)	50	70	85	100
18 × 24		35	17.6	12	9
24 × 30		58	29	20	15

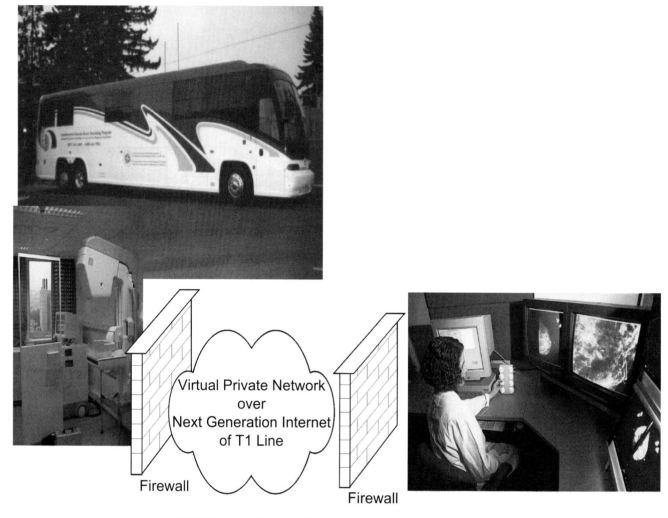

FIGURE 10-1. Schematic diagram of a telemammography system.

examinations. Provisions, such as data encryption and authentication, must be provided to ensure confidentiality of medical data and access only to authorized individuals. Security can be provided by creating virtual private networks for image transmission and by protecting each institution's computer system with a firewall.

For a telemammography system to be practical, its throughput must be sufficiently high that it does not impede workflow. Required speeds depend on the size of the images, the number of images that must be handled per hour and per day, and on how the images will be read. A variety of technologies can be considered for data transmission, including DSL (digital subscriber lines) provided by the telephone company, fiber optic links, high-speed (next generation) Internet, or satellite. These vary in bandwidth (image transmission speed) and cost. Some transmission protocols are given in Table 10-2.

Consider a small mammography facility with a single machine. With a T1 connection, it would require approximately 3 minutes to transmit the data for the four 9-MB

images from a single examination. For consulting purposes, this would be quite feasible and would allow interaction in real time. For a workload of 15 examinations per day, this would generate approximately 540 MB per day.

For larger images (45 MB), these values would all be increased by a factor of 5. Consulting could still be carried

TABLE 10-2. SPEEDS IN MB/S OF SOME CURRENTLY AVAILABLE DATA TRANSMISSION PROTOCOLS

Protocol	Data rate MB/s
56 K FAX modem	.007
DSL	.12
T1	.193
OC3	19.375
OC12	77.75
100 base T	12.5
NGI	125
State-of-the-art (2003)	1250

out with little or no time delay from the patient examination until the images were available for interpretation at the receiving end. Alternatively, a faster communications link could be used.

For a busy facility with four units, each carrying out 25 examinations per day with 45-MB images, the data produced per day would be 18 GB. At T1 rates, this would require 25.9 hours, so that even with full time transmission and no overhead, it would not be possible to transmit this load. On the other hand, with an OC3 network (19.375 MB/s), these images could be sent in just over 15 minutes of transmission time.

Compression

Of course, it is possible to reduce transmission time through image compression. There are two types of compression, lossless and lossy. In lossless compression, whatever operations have been taken to reduce the amount of data to be transmitted can be reversed *exactly*, without any errors. Examples of lossless compression are removal of areas of the image, such as the background, where there is no useful information, and the use of shorthand to describe areas that are uniform. With lossless compression, mammograms can be reduced in size by a factor of 3–6, depending on the size of the breast (1–3).

In lossy compression, operations are undertaken that could affect restoration of the restored image, so that it might differ in minor ways from the precompressed original. Compression factors of 20:1 or more could be achieved using modern lossy compression methods, probably without any diagnostic significance. Nevertheless, for medicolegal reasons, lossy compression might not be acceptable in mammography.

It is important to recognize that image transmission times may not be the only bottleneck in telemammography. For a system to be practical, the routing and loading of images must be fast and preferably automatic. In general, both in telemammography and in normal softcopy display, the need for manual computer operations to access, load, or manipulate images must be kept to a minimum.

Potential for Telemammography

Sickles has demonstrated that expert mammographers interpreting digital images sent by telemammography and viewed on softcopy perform with greater accuracy than general radiologists viewing the original images. However, he has also pointed out that for telemammography to be practical and cost effective, it is necessary to be able to do softcopy image interpretation (4). This is now the case with the smaller image formats; however, softcopy workstations that are user friendly are only beginning to emerge for the highest resolution digital mammography systems.

The potential for telemammography is enormous. It would allow interpretation of mammograms by radiologists with the greatest expertise, and it would use the radiologist's time more efficiently. In the future, it could allow consultation on difficult cases with experts anywhere in the world. Within an institution, it would provide better and more efficient communication among radiologists, surgeons, and oncologists. The use of computer or telephone voice communication and synchronized cursors on the displays at the sending and receiving stations would allow interaction among these individuals in a manner similar to their working together in the same room. The National Library of Medicine has been supporting the development of a National Digital Mammography Archive which uses telemammography over the Next Generation Internet (5). It includes distributed archiving to connect facilities nationally or internationally. This would make practical the retrieval of previous examinations from facilities in other cities or countries.

One exciting application that could bring high-quality mammography to women in very sparsely populated areas is mobile digital mammography, transported on a bus or a small aircraft. An experienced mammographic technologist would travel with the unit, visiting remote communities. Digital mammograms from either screening or diagnostic examinations could then be transmitted to a center with experts for remote interpretation. One of the challenges with this application is to have a high-speed, affordable communications link to the mobile unit. Recent developments in wireless digital communication might help solve this problem. Another possibility is the combination of telemammography with CAD to help make this tool more accessible and more cost effective for small and remote facilities.

TOMOSYNTHESIS

Digital mammography provides images with improved dynamic range and SNR, as well as the ability to adjust image brightness and contrast after acquisition. Despite these improvements, digital mammography, like its predecessor, is often limited because the shadows of structures within the volume of the breast are superimposed when projected onto the two-dimensional image receptor. The resulting densities can mask the presence of lesions or can simulate a lesion when none exists. One can consider the density in the mammogram due to objects in the breast above and below the plane containing an object of interest as a form of structural noise.

Conventional and computed tomography (CT) have demonstrated the advantages of simplifying images by removing the effects of superimposition and presenting the image as a set of slices to convey the three-dimensional arrangement of tissue structures. Digital mammography presents an opportunity to achieve similar advantages through tomosynthesis.

Tomosynthesis is similar to tomography in that the image is acquired by moving the x-ray source during the exposure time. In linear tomography, the path of the source is that of a straight line above the breast. In tomography, the image receptor is also moved linearly in the opposite direction during a continuous x-ray exposure. The motion is designed so that structures in a particular plane, containing the fulcrum or pivot of the motion, are projected onto the same location in the image regardless of the position of the x-ray source and receptor. Structures in other planes are projected onto a range of locations causing them to be blurred. The amount of blurring is greater as the distance from the fulcrum plane increases. In linear tomography, this blurring takes place in only one direction—that of the motion of the source and receptor.

In tomosynthesis, the digital detector remains stationary, and only the x-ray source is moved. Rather than a continuous exposure, a number of individual stationary digital images are acquired, one at each angle of the x-ray source. A system for breast tomosynthesis was developed by Niklason and his colleagues (6). It was designed around the geometry of a conventional digital mammography system. In addition to the usual gantry motions required for mammographic positioning, an additional rotation of the arm holding the x-ray tube is provided. To accommodate the wider range of angular incidence of x-rays on the detector,

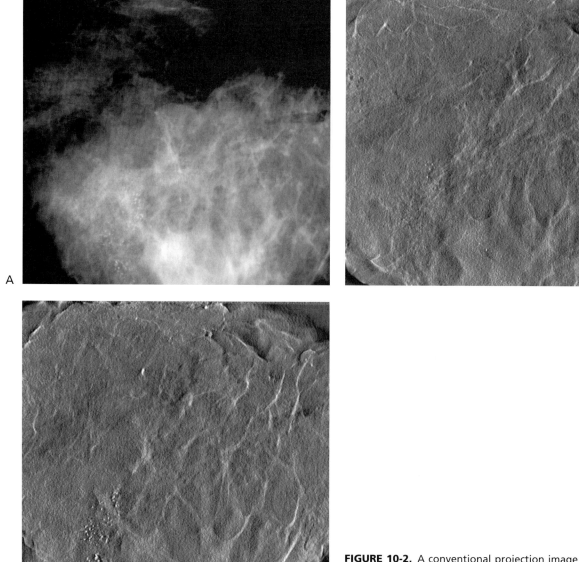

FIGURE 10-2. A conventional projection image of breast tissue containing microcalcifications **(A)** and tomosynthetic images of two different slices, illustrating the three-dimensional arrangement of the calcifications **(B,C)**. (Courtesy Dr. L. Niklason.)

no antiscatter grid is employed. Otherwise, x-rays entering at large angles from the normal to the detector would be absorbed by the grid septa.

The trajectory of the x-ray source in this configuration is an arc rather than a line. Image data can be transformed to simulate a straight-line path of the source across the breast. The individual digital images are shifted an appropriate amount to simulate the motion of the receptor and added appropriately to produce images of a series of slices through the breast. Figure 2 illustrates a conventional projection image of breast tissue containing microcalcifications and two separate tomosynthetic slices (6). Whereas in the conventional image, all of the calcifications are superimposed, the tomosynthetic images provide a better indication of their three-dimensional arrangement within the breast.

Because the acquisition is in digital form, the exposure employed per angular view can be very small. The effect of combining multiple views increases the effective SNR. In the series from which Figure 10-2 was taken, 11 images were obtained with a total dose to the breast just slightly higher than that which would be received from one conventional digital mammogram.

Because the data for tomosynthesis are acquired at multiple angles, with the source and detector stationary during each x-ray exposure, the out-of-slice structures are not blurred, but merely shifted, as is illustrated in Figure 10-3. The effect is that the contrast of structures in the focal plane is reinforced, while that of out-of-slice tissue is diluted (Fig. 10-4). It is possible to apply filtering operations to reduce the effects of out-of-slice structures on the image (7,8). The more angles at which images are acquired, the greater will be the contrast advantage of the structures in the focal plane. Future developments in tomosynthesis will include optimization of filtering techniques to reduce contributions from out-of-plane tissue. In addition, multiaxial motion can be used to remove the effects of out-of-plane tissue more uniformly.

CONTRAST DIGITAL MAMMOGRAPHY

Current digital mammography (CDM) has high sensitivity and specificity in detecting breast cancer, particularly when microcalcifications are present and the arrangement of fat and fibroglandular tissue provides adequate contrast to allow the depiction of masses, architectural distortion, or asymmetry. The accuracy of mammography tends to decrease in dense breasts, where lesions are often surrounded by fibroglandular tissue, which reduces their conspicuity. Even when lesions are detected, the full extent of disease may not be clearly presented.

It has been shown that the growth and metastatic potential of tumors can be directly linked to the extent of surrounding angiogenesis (9). These new vessels proliferate in a disorganized manner and are of poor quality. This makes them leaky and causes blood to pool around the tumor. This motivates the use of contrast medium uptake imaging methods to aid in the detection and diagnosis of cancer.

Contrast-enhanced breast MRI using the gadolinium based contrast agent, Gd-DTPA, has shown high sensitivity and moderate specificity in the detection of breast cancer (10–15). Heywang-Köbrunner and others found that malignant tumors tend to enhance rapidly, reaching their peak enhancement within one or two minutes, as opposed to benign tumors that enhance much more slowly, reaching their peak enhancement after many minutes. The drawbacks with contrast-enhanced MRI, however, are that it is time consuming and costly.

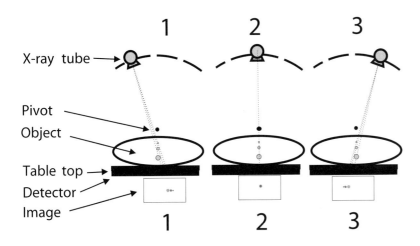

FIGURE 10-3. Schematic of tomosynthesis. A series of digital radiographs is acquired as the tube moves on an arc about the pivot point. The detector remains stationary and is read out after each exposure.

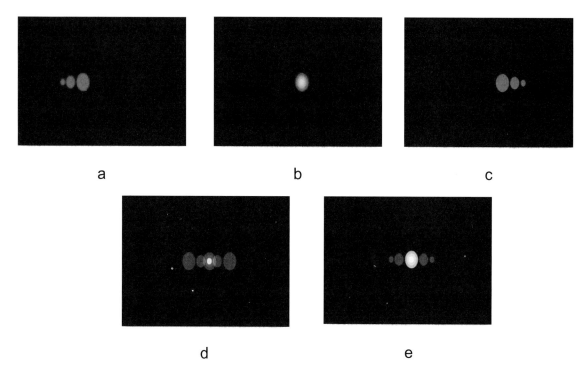

a   b   c

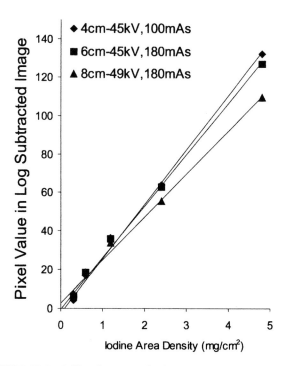

d   e

FIGURE 10-4. (A–E) Reconstruction of tomosynthetic slices in different planes by shifting and adding digital image data. **(A–C)** Projections at positions 1, 2, 3 respectively. **(D,E)** Reconstructions of uppermost and lowest objects respectively.

The highly improved technology now available in digital mammography encourages an investigation into the use of this modality to perform a contrast-enhanced examination of the breast. We have carried out computer modeling and experimental studies to determine how to optimize the acquisition and processing of contrast digital mammography (CDM) images and to understand the attainable contrast sensitivity of the technique (16). A digital mammography system can be calibrated to provide quantitative measurements of the projected concentration (in mg/cm²) of iodine along a ray path through the breast (Fig. 10-5).

A pilot investigation was carried out with patients who had suspicious lesions that were initially detected on conventional mammography and who were scheduled to receive either core needle biopsy or excisional biopsy (17). The contrast agent used for this study was nonionic iodine (Omnipaque 300 iohexol).

At energies above iodine's k-edge (33.2keV), the difference in attenuation between iodine and breast tissue is maximized. Therefore, x-rays at these energies will create the largest possible contrast between iodine and breast tissue in the acquired image. To shape the x-ray spectrum so as to maximize the proportion of x-rays that have energies above 33.2keV, the molybdenum target mammography tube of a GE 2000D digital mammography system was operated at 49 kV, and the beam was filtered with copper.

FIGURE 10-5. Calibration curve for imaging iodine using a digital mammography system and subtraction imaging. Concentrations as low as 0.3 mg cm² can be measured. Curves depend on breast thickness and kV because of scattering and beam hardening effects.

The breast is lightly compressed, with enough pressure to limit motion of the breast, but not enough to reduce blood flow significantly. First, a single "mask" image is produced. Immediately following this exposure, the women were injected in the antecubital vein with 75–100mL of Omnipaque 300 iohexol. A series of approximately 5 postcontrast images is then acquired over 7–10 minutes.

The precontrast mask image and the postcontrast images are carefully registered to correct as much as possible for the effects of motion between each image acquisition. Next, a logarithmic transform is applied to the mask image and all subsequent postcontrast images. The processed mask image is then subtracted from each of the postcontrast images. In the resulting set of images, any uptake of iodine appears as a white "blush" or a region with higher pixel values than the surrounding tissue.

In our pilot study in which 21 patients were imaged, 8 of the 10 malignant cases and 5 of the 12 benign cases showed enhancement. One of the malignancies that did not enhance was a case of ductal carcinoma in situ (DCIS). The other was a low-grade infiltrating ductal carcinoma. Morphologically, two of the malignancies showed a rim-like appearance (Fig. 10-6). The kinetics of this case followed the pattern frequently seen in malignant lesions on MRI, where there is early uptake of contrast agent (1

min) followed by rapid washout. One case that was infiltrating ductal carcinoma (IDC) with DCIS showed inhomogeneous enhancement with linear areas of enhancement (Fig. 10-7).

In our limited early work, the enhancement kinetics were not sufficiently consistent to allow reliable differentiation of benign from malignant lesions. It is generally believed that for good specificity in breast magnetic resonance imaging (MRI), both morphology and kinetics should be considered. Our results also support this conclusion for CDM.

In our study, enhancement was observed in 89% (8 of 9) of the invasive cancers (PPV = 62%). There was no enhancement in 7 of the 12 benign lesions (58%) that were initially considered worrisome on mammography or ultrasound (NPV 78%). Three cases positive on ultrasound and negative on mammography that did not show enhancement were confirmed to be benign. The morphology of the lesions was generally consistent with the benign and malignant features seen on other imaging modalities.

Possible roles for this technique are similar to those for breast MRI, that is, detection of lesions not clearly seen on mammography and improved delineation of extent of disease. Now that the technique has demonstrated the ability to show cancers, we plan to recruit women with dense breasts and mammographically occult or subtle findings to evaluate the possible additional benefit over regular mammography.

Lewin and colleagues have discussed a dual-energy approach to contrast digital mammography and have showed images similar to those presented here. In this technique, two images are produced in rapid sequence, one con-

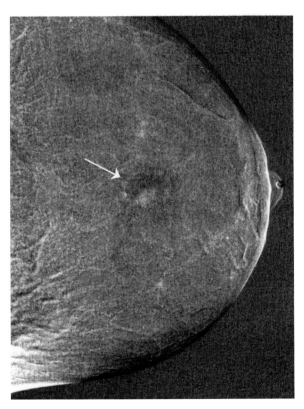

FIGURE 10-6. Subtraction digital mammogram of an invasive tumor (*arrow*) showing rim enhancement.

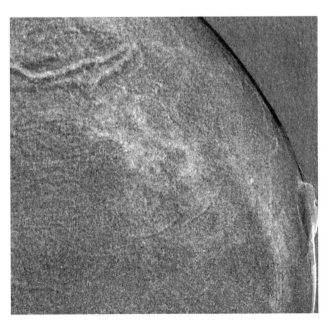

FIGURE 10-7. Subtraction image of invasive ductal carcinoma with ductal carcinoma in situ.

taining x-rays predominantly below the k-edge of iodine (33.2 keV) and one at higher energy. The iodine signal is isolated by performing a weighted subtraction of the two images. This procedure eliminates the need to produce a mask image, thereby minimizing the effects of motion between the two images.

Another possible area for improvement is the elimination of background uptake from overlying and underlying tissues in the breast. With even a low level of uptake in these superimposed and adjacent tissues, the projected signal of the entire thickness of the breast could reduce the conspicuity of a lesion and affect the quantitative measurements. This problem with overlying tissue does not occur with breast MRI, which produces tomographic images. With CDM, the problem could be overcome by combining it with a tomographic technique such as tomosynthesis

The results of this preliminary study suggest that CDM may be potentially useful in identifying lesions in the mammographically dense breast. As in MRI, other applications may be useful in identifying the extent of disease or detecting an otherwise occult carcinoma that has presented with axillary metastases. This information may aid in the diagnosis and guidance of core biopsy or excision of these lesions. CDM may also be helpful in monitoring response to neoadjuvant and antiangiogenic therapy.

With the increasing availability of digital mammography, CDM will become accessible and relatively inexpensive compared to current MRI technology. These results encourage further investigation of CDM as a diagnostic tool for breast cancer.

MEASUREMENT OF MAMMOGRAPHIC DENSITY FOR RISK ASSESSMENT

In our work, it is very useful to digitize film mammograms and calculate *mammographic density* of the images. Mammographic density refers loosely to the proportion of the image that corresponds to fibroglandular tissue as opposed to fat. Wolfe suggested that there was a relationship between density, which he characterized in terms of *parenchymal patterns,* and risk of future breast cancer (18). This association has been verified by several others who have assessed density using a variety of qualitative and quantitative methods (19–22). In our work, an interactive thresholding method is used to measure the fractional area of the mammogram that is dense (23). The user interface for the software created to facilitate these measurements is shown in Figure 10-8. It allows adjustment of brightness and contrast of the display to demonstrate the skin line and the parenchymal and stromal features of the breast. While viewing the image, the user adjusts a threshold control. All pixels whose value is the same as the threshold setting are illuminated in color. The threshold is set to correspond to the value that distinguishes the image of the breast from the surrounding background. Then a second threshold is chosen to segment the dense (i.e., brighter) regions from the more fatty regions in the image. Once the thresholds have been established, all of the pixels in the image of the breast can be counted to obtain its area. The area of dense pixels is also determined from those pixels with values above the second threshold. Then, the ratio of these areas or fractional

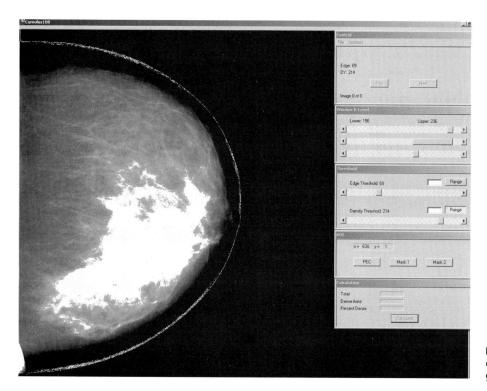

FIGURE 10-8. Software tool for two-dimensional assessment of mammographic density.

density is calculated. We have shown that for women whose breasts contain greater than 75% dense tissue by area, there is a 4- to 6-fold increased risk compared to those whose density is less than breasts that are fatty replaced (24). Thus, breast density is one of the strongest predictors of breast cancer risk.

It is reasonable that the mechanism for breast cancer risk should be more closely related to the actual volume of dense tissue rather than its projected area. Therefore, we have been working to develop a method for determining volumetric density. This can be done by calibrating the mammography system so that the brightness information in the image has quantitative meaning. In Figure 10-9A is shown a step wedge, varying in thickness from 0 to 8 cm in one direction. In the other direction, along each step, the composition of a tissue-equivalent plastic is varied from being equivalent to the x-ray attenuation of fat to that of 100% fibroglandular tissue.

From the digitized image of the step wedge, a surface like that of Figure 10-9B can be developed where there is a relationship among image brightness (radiation absorbed by the screen), breast thickness, and composition. Therefore, if breast thickness is accurately known, the composition can be determined for the path through the breast corresponding to each image pixel from the recorded signal. It is then possible to determine the volume of dense tissue, the total breast volume, and the ratio between them (i.e., the volumetric breast density) (25).

This type of information could have several uses. By predicting a woman's risk of breast cancer, it might be possible to develop an optimized strategy for breast cancer surveillance, employing the most appropriate frequency of various imaging modalities for screening. For example, women at the highest risk might be screened with breast MRI. In the short term, as a surrogate marker for risk, mammographic density can be used in studies to investigate etiologic factors for breast cancer, which may include genetic factors, diet, use of medications, and lifestyle (26–30). In the case where a potential risk-reducing strategy is available, changes in mammographic density might be used as an early indicator of response.

One of the limitations of screen-film mammography is the difficulty of extracting quantitative information from the images. To do this, it is necessary to scan and digitize the film. This is time consuming and expensive. There is also loss of information both from the digitization process and because of the basic limitations of the quality of information on the original film because of its limited dynamic range and SNR.

With digital mammography, it is straightforward to obtain quantitative data from the images simply by accessing the DICOM file. The wide dynamic range of the detectors and the methods for self-calibration of the system should provide high stability that facilitates quantitative use of data from digital mammography. It is important, however, to realize that the data do undergo various stages of

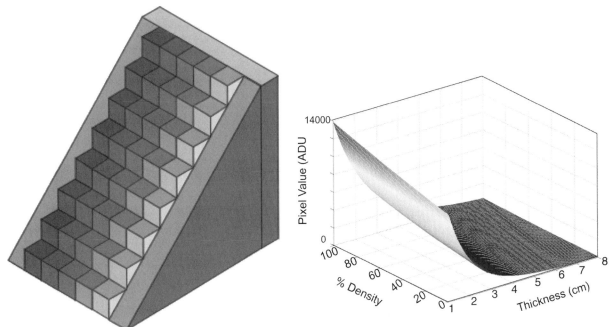

A   B

FIGURE 10-9. (A) Calibration device for determination of volumetric density. **(B)** Calibration surface for volumetric density. From the measurement of x-ray transmission provided by the digital system and knowledge of the breast thickness, the composition (fraction fibroglandular) corresponding to each pixel can be determined.

processing. Usually the earliest stage at which the data are accessible to the user is after correction for dark signal and gain variation from del to del has been performed. This is often referred to as the "raw" image. At this point, the pixel values in the image are proportional to the amount of x-ray energy that has been absorbed in the detector element(s) corresponding to that pixel, which, in turn, is related to the x-ray transmission through the breast. This proportionality is most cases linear. In the case of the Fuji photostimulable system, however, it is logarithmic. Digital mammography systems often apply further image processing operations, such as linear or nonlinear scaling, peripheral thickness equalization, and artifact removal before the processed image is provided to the user. Therefore, it is important to have a clear idea of what transformations are applied to the data before attempting to use them quantitatively.

REFERENCES

1. National Electrical Manufacturer's Association (NEMA) DICOM Standards Committee, Working Group 15. Digital Mammography. Digital Imaging and Communication in Medicine. http://medical.nema.org
2. Lou SL, Sickles EA, Huang HK, et al. Full-field direct digital telemammography: technical components, study protocols, and preliminary results. IEEE Trans Inf Technol Biomed 1997;1: 270–278.
3. Huang HK, Lou SL. Telemammography: A technical overview. In: Haus AG, Yaffe MJ, eds. Physical Aspects of Breast Imaging: Current and Future Considerations. RSNA Publications, 1999: 273-281.
4. Sickles EA. Computer-aided diagnosis and telemammography: Clinical perspective. In: Haus AG, Yaffe MJ, eds. Physical Aspects of Breast Imaging: Current and Future Considerations. RSNA Publications, 1999:283–285.
5. Beckerman BG, Batsell SG, MacIntyre LP, et al. Feasibility of telemammography as biomedical application for breast imaging. In: Vo-Dinh T, Grundfest WA, Benaron DA, Charles ST, Bucholz RD, Vannier MW, eds. Biomedical Diagnostic, Guidance, and Surgical-Assist Systems. SPIE Proc 1999;3595:49–60.
6. Niklason LT, Christian BT, Niklason LE, et al. Digital tomosynthesis in breast imaging. Radiology 1997;205:399–406.
7. Kolitsi Z, Panayiotakis G, Pallikarakis N. A method for selective removal of out-of-plane structures in digital tomosynthesis. Med Phys 1993;20(1):47–50.
8. Webber RL, Underhill HR, Freimanis RI. Evaluation of observer performance of spot mammograms obtained from a hybrid breast phantom using tuned-aperture computed tomography and standardized controls. In: Yaffe MJ, ed. IWDM 2000 5th International Workshop on Digital Mammography. Toronto, ON: Medical Physics Publishing, 2000:102–107.
9. Weidner N, Semple JP, Welch WR, et al. Tumor angiogenesis and metastasis correlation in invasive breast carcinoma. N Engl J Med 1991;324:1–7.
10. Heywang S, Wolf A, Pruss E, et al. MR imaging of the breast with Gd-DTPA: Use and limitations. Radiology 1989;171: 95–103.
11. Heywang-Köbrunner S. Contrast-enhanced magnetic resonance imaging of the breast. Investigative Radiology 1994;29:94–104.
12. Kaiser WA, Zeitler E. MR imaging of the breast: fast imaging sequence with and without Gd-DTPA preliminary observations. Radiology 1989;170:639–649.
13. Weinreb JC, Newstead G. MR imaging of the breast. Radiology 1995;196;593–610.
14. Harms SE, Flamig DP, Helsey KL, et al. MR imaging of the breast with rotating delivery of excitation off resonance: clinical experience with pathologic correlation. Radiology 1993;187; 493–501.
15. Orel SG, Schnall MD, LiVolsi VA, et al. Suspicious breast lesions: MR imaging with radiology-pathologic correlation. Radiology 1994;190;485–493.
16. Skarpathiotakis M, Yaffe MJ, Bloomquist AK, et al. Development of contrast digital mammography. Med Phys 1002;29 (10):2419–2426.
17. Jong RA, Yaffe MJ, Skarpathiotakis M, et al. Contrast digital mammography: Initial clinical experience (accepted for publication). Radiology 2003.
18. Wolfe JN. Risk for breast cancer development determined by mammographic parenchymal pattern. Cancer 1976;37:2486–2492.
19. Boyd NF, O'Sullivan B, Campbell JE, et al. Mammographic signs as risk factors for breast cancer. Br J Cancer 1982;45:185–193.
20. Brisson J, Verreault R, Morrison A, et al. Diet, mammographic features of breast tissue, and breast cancer risk. Am J Epidemiol 1989;130:14–24.
21. Warner E, Lockwood G, Math M, et al. The risk of breast cancer associated with mammographic parenchymal patterns: A meta-analysis of the published literature to examine the effect of method of classification. Cancer Detect Prev 1992;16:67–72.
22. Byrne C, Schairer C, Wolfe J, et al. Mammographic features and breast cancer risk: effects with time, age, and menopause status, J NCI 1995;87:1622–1629.
23. Byng JW, Boyd NF, Fishell E, et al. The quantitative analysis of mammographic densities. Phys Med Biol 1994;39:1629–1638.
24. Boyd, NF, Byng, JW, Jong, RA, et al. Quantitative classification of mammographic densities and breast cancer risk: Results from the Canadian National Breast Screening Study. J NCI 1995; 87:670–675.
25. Pawluczyk O, Augustine BJ, Yaffe MJ, et al. A volumetric method for estimation of breast density on digitized screen-film mammograms. Med Phys 2003;30:352–364.
26. Boyd NF, Dite GS, Stone J, et al. Heritability of mammographic density: A risk factor for breast cancer. N Engl J Med 2002;347 (12):886–894.
27. Nayfield SG, Karp JE, Ford LG, et al. Potential role of tamoxifen in prevention of breast cancer. J NCI 1991;83:1450–1459.
28. Laya MB, Gallagher JC, Schreiman JS, et al. Effect of postmenopausal hormonal replacement therapy on mammographic density and parenchymal pattern. Radiology 1995;196: 433–437.
29. Boyd NF, Greenberg C, Lockwood G, et al. The effects at 2 years of a low-fat high-carbohydrate diet on radiological features of the breast: Results from a randomized trial. J NCI 1997;89: 488–496.
30. Kaufhold J, Thomas JA, Eberhard JW, et al. Tissue composition determination in digital mammography. Radiology 2001;221P: 188.

11

DIGITAL MAMMOGRAPHY CASES WITH MASSES

CHERIE M. KUZMIAK

CASE 1

58-year-old female, research screening study.

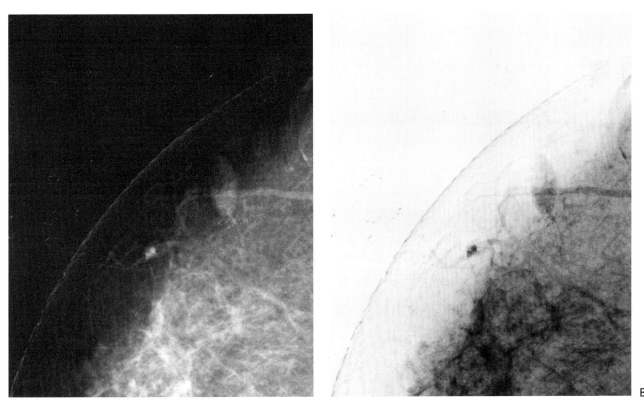

FIGURE 11-1. **(A)** Right breast, CC view enlarged. **(B)** Contrast inverted image of **A**.

Findings

A 1-cm, oval, circumscribed, mixed density mass is present. Its fatty hilum is appreciated in both images.

Conclusion

Intramammary lymph node with a radiolucent center corresponding to the fatty hilum.

Comment

Intramammary lymph nodes can occur in any quadrant of the breast, but are most commonly found in the upper outer quadrant.

If the mass cannot be determined to represent a lymph node on the standard views, then additional views are necessary. Sometimes the inverted image can be helpful in better visualizing the fatty hilum of an intramammary lymph node. Thus, it can prevent the need to expose the patient to additional radiation with extra views. If additional views are not successful, then an ultrasound of the mass may be helpful (as is demonstrated in Case 9).

CASE 2

50-year-old female, research screening study.

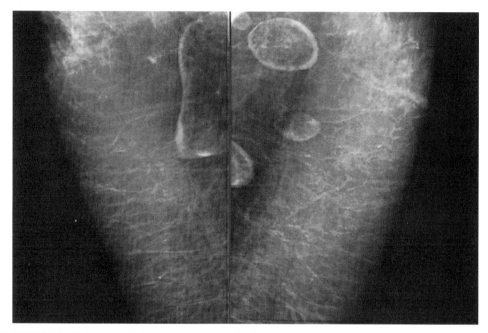

FIGURE 11-2. Right and left breast, MLO views (back to back) with attention to the axillary regions.

Findings

Mixed density masses of varying sizes are visualized in the axillary regions.

Conclusion

Normal lymph nodes.

Comment

Lymph nodes should be considered normal, regardless of size, when a fatty hilum and a symmetric cortex are present.

CASE 3

39-year-old, postpartum female with a palpable right breast mass.

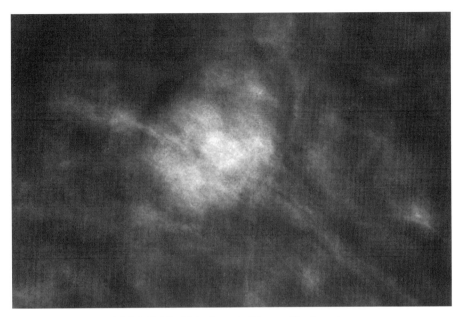

FIGURE 11-3. Right breast, CC magnification view.

Findings

A 1-cm, oval, predominately circumscribed, mixed density mass is present. This corresponds to the area of patient concern.

Conclusion

Galactocele.

Comment

Mixed density masses are benign.

CASE 4

40-year-old female, research screening study.

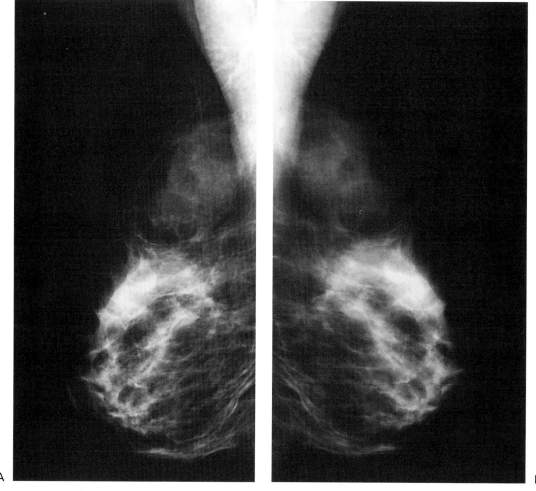

FIGURE 11-4. (A,C) Right breast, MLO and enlarged MLO views, digital. **(B,D)** Right breast, MLO and enlarged MLO views, screen-film. The images are displayed back to back.

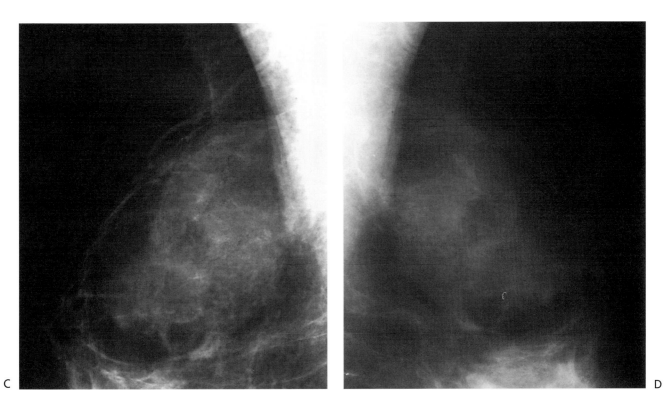

C   D

Findings

A 4-cm oval, mixed-density mass with a capsule is present in the superior aspect of the breast.

Conclusion

Hamartoma (fibroadenolipoma).

Comment

This benign mass, composed of variable amounts of fat, glandular tissue, and fibrous connective tissue is seen with both imaging modalities without difficulty. However, there is increased conspicuity of the capsule on the digital study.

CASE 5

77-year-old female with a subareolar right breast mass.

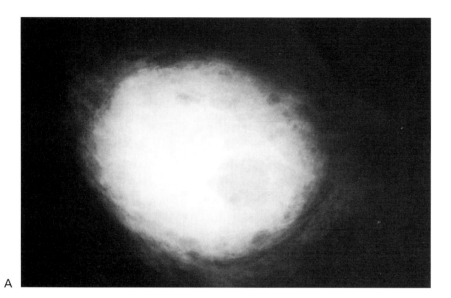

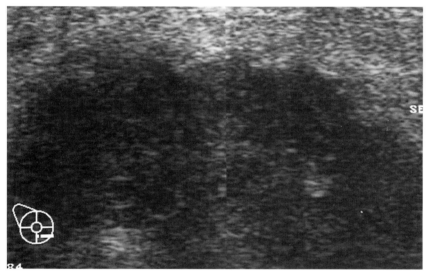

FIGURE 11-5. (A) Right breast, MLO magnification view. **(B)** Ultrasound of the mass.

Findings

A 6-cm × 5-cm, oval, predominately circumscribed, mixed-density mass is present. The ultrasound shows a solid appearing, heterogeneous, irregular mass. The mass is palpable, and the skin above the lesion demonstrated minimal erythema.

Conclusion

Abscess versus inflammatory breast cancer.

Histology

Abscess with acute and chronic inflammation.

Comment

The mixed density was secondary to a previous fine needle aspiration performed by a surgeon. The lucency represents air. The mass is an abscess. The patient was treated surgically, and had an uncomplicated recovery.

CASE 6

40-year-old female, asymptomatic.

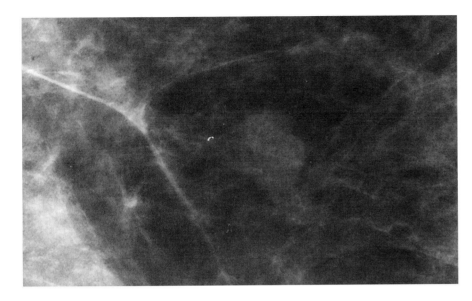

FIGURE 11-6. Right breast, CC magnification view.

Findings

A 1-cm, oval, lobulated, predominately circumscribed, low-density mass, without associated features, is seen. The anterior border is obscured. Benign type calcifications are present anterior to the mass.

The mass was a simple cyst sonographically.

Conclusion

Benign mass.

Comment

Not only it is important to characterize a mass by its size, shape, margins, and associated features, but it is also important to characterize its density. The density of a mass is based on the comparison of its overall "whiteness" (ability to attenuate photons) when compared to the normal breast parenchyma.

Low-density masses are almost always benign. Masses that are of equal density to the tissue are usually benign. High-density masses have a higher probability of being malignant. Nevertheless, when a lesion is evaluated it should be classified by its most worrisome features.

CASE 7

43-year-old female, history of cysts.

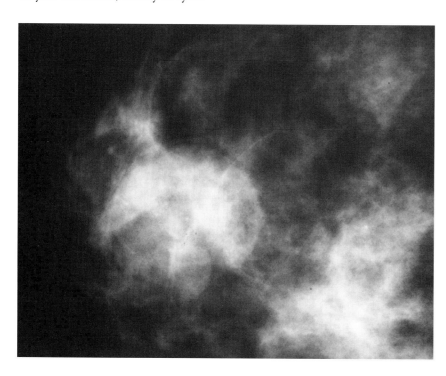

FIGURE 11-7. Right breast, CC view enlarged.

Findings

A 3-cm, oval, lobulated, circumscribed, isodense mass is present in the subareolar region.

The mass was a simple cyst sonographically.

Conclusion

Mammographically benign mass.

Comment

Ultrasound can be used to determine if a mass is solid or cystic.

CASE 8

58-year-old-female, research screening study.

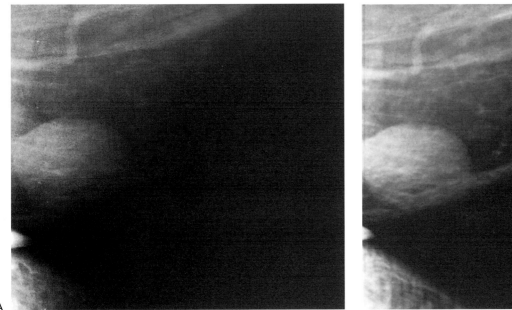

A   B

FIGURE 11-8. (A) Left breast, CC view enlarged, screen-film. **(B)** Left breast, CC view enlarged, digital.

Findings

A 1-cm, circumscribed, isodense mass is seen in the medial aspect of the breast within the subcutaneous tissue. The digital image displays the skin line and subcutaneous tissue better than the film-screen study.

Sonographically, the mass was hypoechoic and located in the subcutaneous tissue.

Conclusion

Sebaceous cyst.

Comment

Sebaceous cysts are commonly found in the cleavage and axillary regions, but can be located anywhere in the skin.

CASE 9

70-year-old female with a painful left breast.

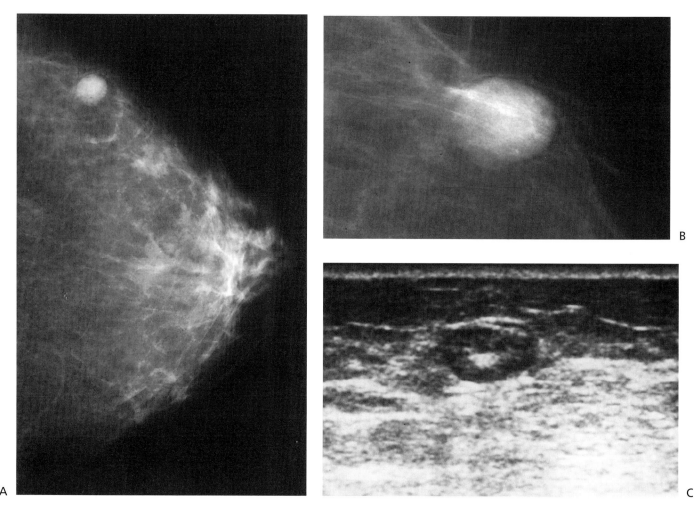

FIGURE 11-9. **(A)** Left breast, CC view. **(B)** CC magnification view. **(C)** Ultrasound of the mass.

Findings

A 1.5-cm, oval, circumscribed, isodense mass is noted in the lateral aspect of the breast.
No definite fatty hilum is identified. The mass is not palpable.

Sonographically, the mass is seen to be a normal lymph node with a fatty hilum.

Conclusion

Intramammary lymph node.

Comment

Breast fat is hypoechoic with ultrasound, unlike fat in the rest of the body which is hyperechoic.

The fatty hilum of a lymph node is hyperechoic.

CASE 10

55-year-old female with a palpable subareolar right breast mass and a history of clear spontaneous nipple discharge from that breast.

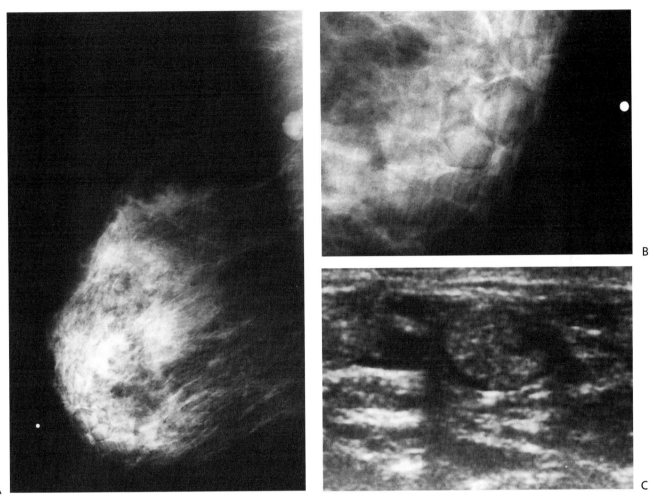

FIGURE 11-10. (A) Right breast, MLO view. A metallic BB marks the area of concern. **(B)** MLO magnification view. The images are displayed back to back. **(C)** Ultrasound of one of the subareolar masses.

Findings

Three oval, circumscribed, isodense masses are seen in the subareolar region. Mammographically these masses are benign.

They represent intraductal masses with ultrasound. One of the masses is seen in a dilated duct with ultrasound in Figure 11-10C. A surgical excision was performed.

Histology

Intraductal papillomas.

Comment

A papilloma is a benign hyperplastic growth with a central fibrovascular core that is usually located in a major duct in the breast. They can be multiple. Papilloma's most frequently present as a spontaneous sanguineous/serous nipple discharge or with a palpable subareolar mass. Mammography usually shows no findings or with a subareolar mass with or without calcifications, or less frequently, calcifications only.

When a patient has spontaneous sanguineous/serous nipple discharge with no mammographic finding on the standard views, magnification views of the subareolar region and ultrasound of the symptomatic side are recommended for further evaluation. Ductography may also be performed if the additional views and ultrasound are unremarkable.

CASE 11

50 year-old female with a left breast mass.

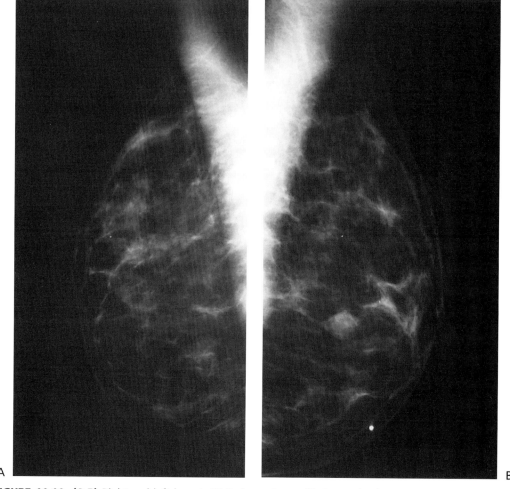

A

B

FIGURE 11-11. (A,B) Right and left breast, MLO views. A metallic BB marks the area of concern. **(C)** MLO magnification view. **(D)** Left breast ultrasound.

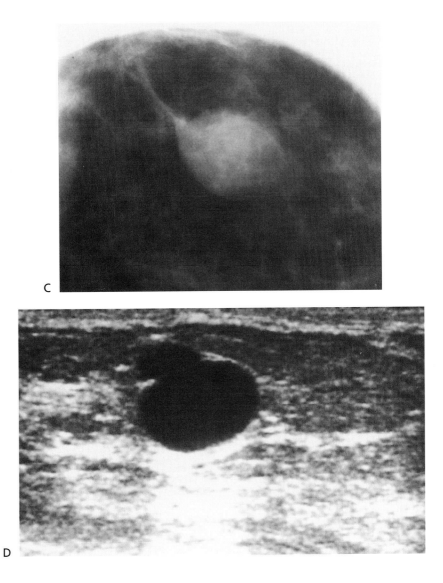

C

D

Findings

A 1.5-cm, oval, circumscribed, isodense mass is present in the central subareolar region of the left breast.

The mass represents two adjacent cysts sonographically. The areas of patient concern inferiorly represents normal fat lobules.

Conclusion

Benign masses.

CASE 12

50 year-old-female, research screening study.

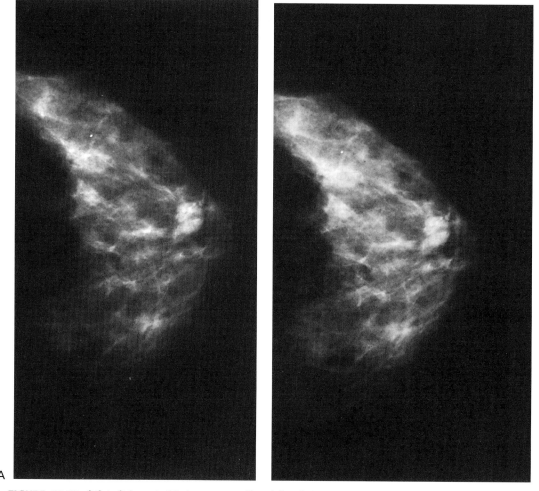

A   B

FIGURE 11-12. (A) Left breast, CC view, screen-film. **(B)** Left breast, CC view, digital. **(C)** CC magnification view, digital. **(D)** Ultrasound of the mass.

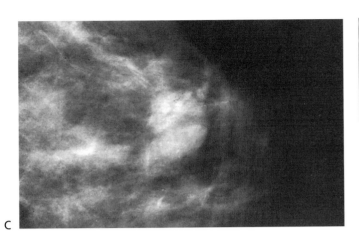

C

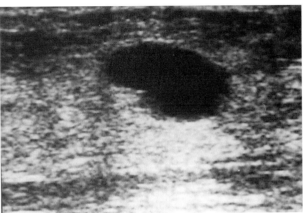

D

Findings

A 1.5-cm, oval mass and benign type calcifications are present in the subareolar region. The margins of the mass are both circumscribed and obscured.

The mass is a simple cyst with ultrasound.

Comment

Both digital and screen-film mammography equally demonstrate this mass.

CASE 13

38-year-old female, history of polycystic ovarian disease.

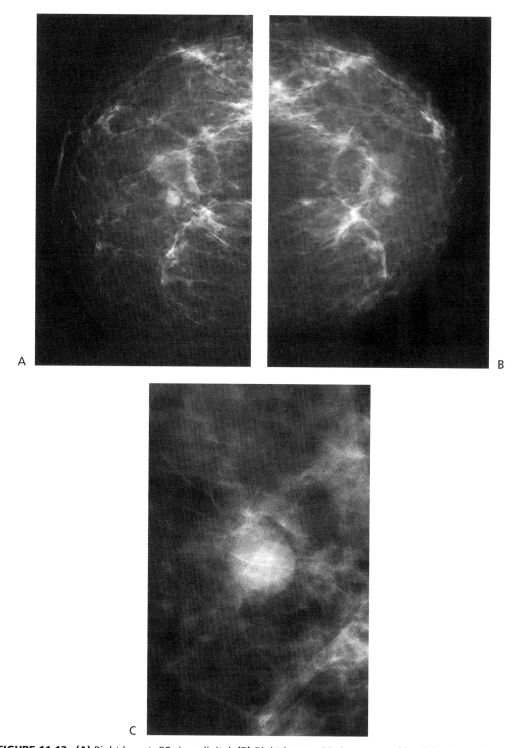

FIGURE 11-13. (A) Right breast, CC view, digital. **(B)** Right breast, CC view, screen-film. **(C)** CC magnification view, digital. **(D)** Ultrasound of the mass. **(E)** The fibrous stroma is causing compression of the duct epithelium (H&E, 20×).

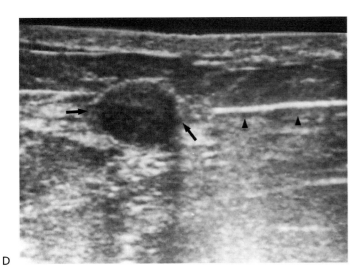

D

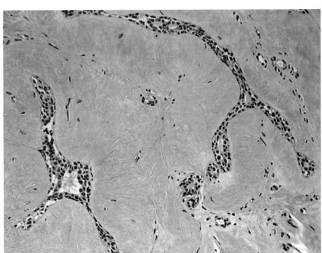

E

Findings

A 1-cm, round, predominately circumscribed, isodense mass is identified in the central subareolar region of the breast, 8-cm from the nipple. The anterior margin of the mass is obscured on the additional magnification image.

Sonographically, the mass is solid, heterogeneous, horizontally oriented, and without posterior shadowing. However, the margins (*arrows*) of the mass are irregular in Figure 11-13D. An ultrasound guided core biopsy was performed. The 14-gauge core biopsy needle is represented by the thick echogenic line (*arrowheads*) in Figure 11-13D.

Histology

Hyalinized fibroadenoma (Fig 11-13E).

Comment

This mass is visualized in the breast with both digital and screen-film mammography.

CASE 14

43-year-old female, asymptomatic.

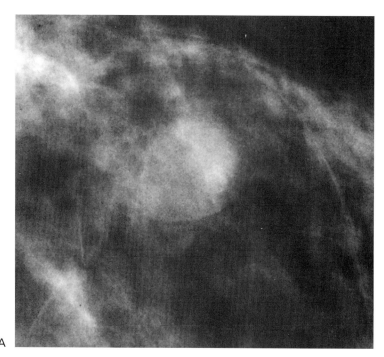

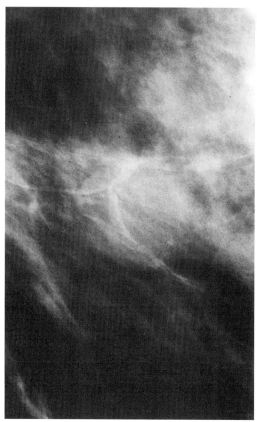

FIGURE 11-14. (A) Left breast, CC magnification view. **(B)** Left breast, MLO magnification view. **(C)** Anastamosing slit-like spaces are seen and are lined by myofibroblasts within a dense collagenous stroma (H&E, 100×).

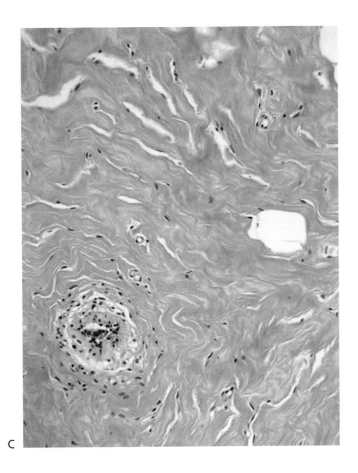

C

Findings

A 1-cm, oval, circumscribed and obscured, isodense mass is demonstrated. This mass was new when compared to a previous study (not shown).

Ultrasound of the mass showed it to be solid, hypoechoic, and horizontally oriented. An ultrasound core biopsy was performed.

Histology

Pseudoangiomatous stromal hyperplasia (Fig. 11-14C).

Comment

Pseudoangiomatous stromal hyperplasia is a benign process. However, it is important for the pathologist to distinguish this entity from the more ominous diagnosis of angiosarcoma.

CASE 15

40-year-old female, history of cysts.

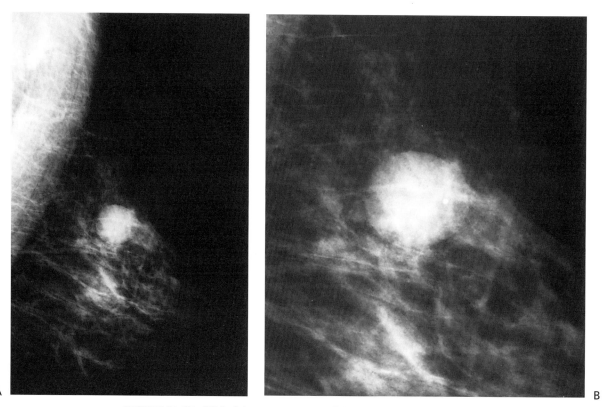

FIGURE 11-15. (A) Left breast, MLO view. **(B)** MLO magnification view.

Findings

A 2-cm, round, circumscribed mass is seen in the superior left breast, 6-cm from the nipple. The overall density appears increased, but this is probably secondary to superimposition with adjacent structures. Notice that along the periphery of the mass, normal breast structures can be seen through it.

Ultrasound showed the mass to be a simple cyst.

Conclusion

Benign mass.

CASE 16

45-year-old female, history of cysts.

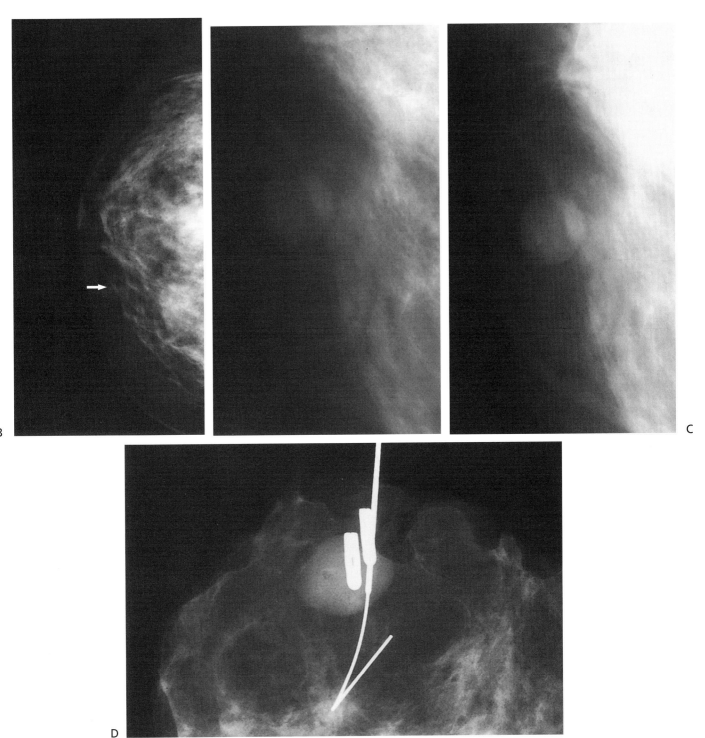

FIGURE 11-16. **(A)** Right breast, CC view. **(B)** CC magnification view. **(C)** Manipulated image of B. **(D)** Specimen radiograph of the mass.

Findings

Multiple, probably benign, oval masses are seen. A 1-cm, oval mass is present in the medial aspect of the breast anteriorly. This is difficult to appreciate on the standard view (*arrow*). The additional views with different windowing and leveling allow this oval, circumscribed, isodense mass to be seen.

The mass was solid by ultrasound. The rest of the masses were simple cysts.
Do to patient anxiety, the solid mass was surgically removed (Fig. 11-16D).

Histology

Fibroadenoma.

Comment

A fibroadenoma is a benign mass composed of varying amounts of fibrous and epithelial elements. It can be very cellular or predominately fibrotic in nature (as is shown in Case 13). Fibroadenomas are more common in young women and are hormonally responsive.

CASE 17

46-year-old female, asymptomatic.

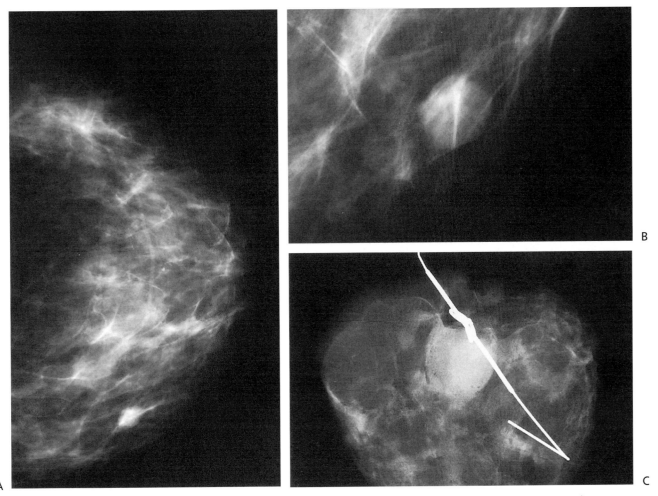

FIGURE 11-17. (A) Left breast, CC view, screen-film. **(B)** CC magnification view, digital. **(C)** Specimen radiograph with the localized mass.

Findings

A 1.5-cm, oval, lobulated mass is visualized in the medial aspect of the breast. Its margins are circumscribed and obscured.

The mass was solid, heterogeneous, and equivocal in orientation by ultrasound. An ultrasound guided core biopsy was performed, and showed fibrocystic changes with atypia. A surgical excision was performed (Fig. 11-17C).

Histology

Fibroadenoma with atypia.

Comment

Because atypia was demonstrated on the core biopsy, a surgical excision was performed.

CASE 18

37-year-old female with a palpable subareolar left breast mass.

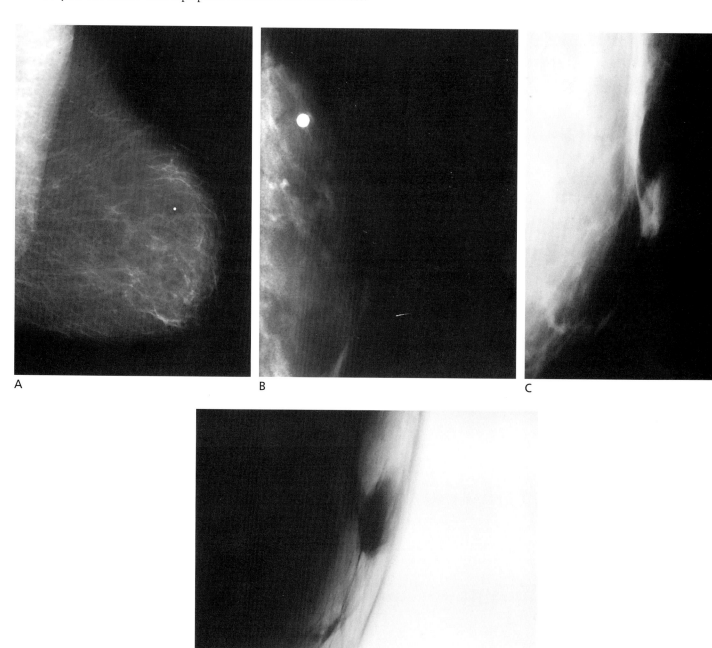

A

B

C

D

FIGURE 11-18. **(A)** Left breast, MLO view, screen-film. **(B)** MLO magnification view, screen-film. **(C,D)** MLO magnification and contrast inverted view, digital. **(E)** Ultrasound of the mass. **(F)** A pericanicular pattern with focal apocrine metaplasia is present (H&E, 20×).

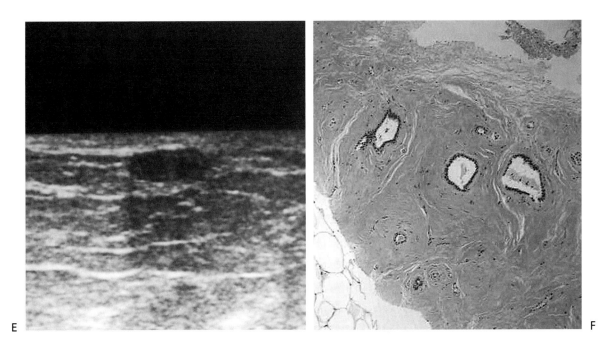

E   F

Findings

No discrete abnormality is seen on the screen-film images.

A 1-cm, oval, circumscribed mass is visualized beneath the skin on the digital images.

The ultrasound demonstrates the mass to be solid and located in the breast tissue (Fig. 11-18E). The patient wanted the mass surgically removed.

Histology

Fibroadenoma (Fig. 11-18F).

Comment

This is an example in which windowing and leveling with the softcopy display system can provide additional information to the radiologist in analyzing a digital mammogram.

CASE 19

75-year-old female, asymptomatic.

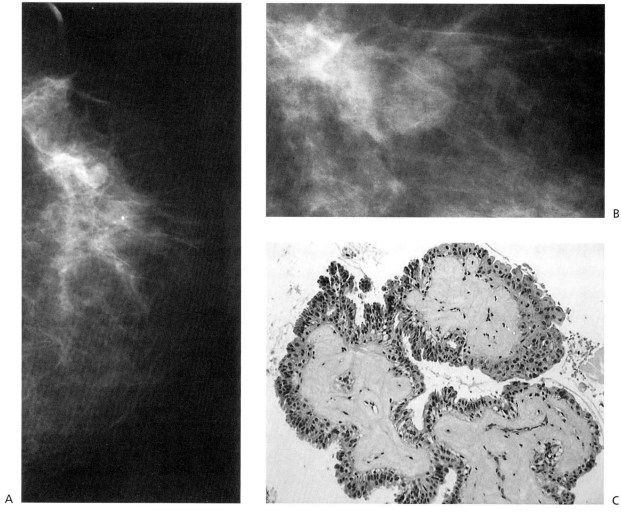

FIGURE 11-19. (A) Left breast, CC view, screen-film. **(B)** CC magnification view, digital. **(C)** Ductal epithelial hyperplasia with papillary architectural and focal nuclear atypia is present (H&E, 40×).

Findings

A 1-cm, oval, isodense mass is identified in the lateral aspect of the breast, 6-cm from the nipple. The margins of the mass are predominately circumscribed.

Sonographically, the mass was solid with irregular margins. An ultrasound guided core biopsy was performed. Histology showed an atypical intraductal papilloma. Since a papillary neoplasm could not be excluded, the mass was surgically removed.

Histology

Intraductal papilloma with atypia (Fig. 11-19C).

CASE 20

45-year-old female, screening research study.

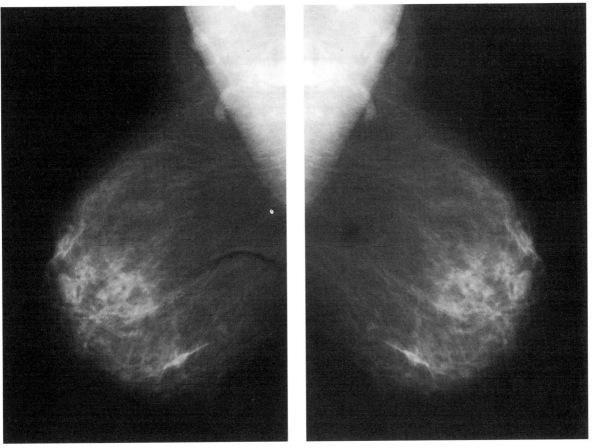

A   B

FIGURE 11-20. (A) Left breast, MLO view, screen-film. **(B)** Left breast, MLO view, digital. **(C,D)** MLO and CC magnification views, digital.

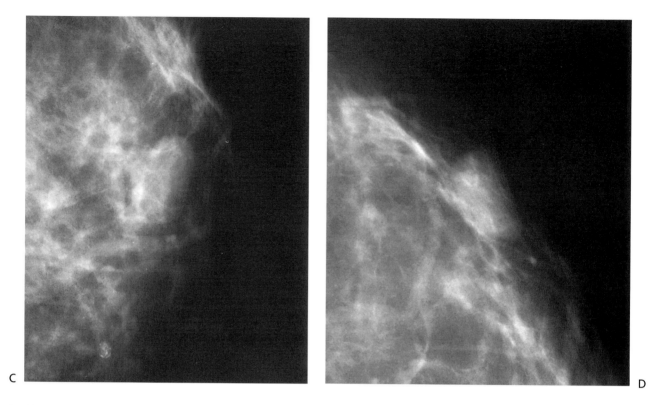

C   D

Findings

A 1.5-cm, oval, circumscribed, isodense mass is present in the subareolar region of the breast. The characteristics of the mass are best seen in the magnification views.

The mass was solid and had benign features sonographically. However, the patient wanted the mass sampled.

Histology

Fibroadenoma.

Comment

The mass is seen clearly with both digital and screen-film mammography.

CASE 21

37-year-old female with a palpable mass at her lumpectomy site.

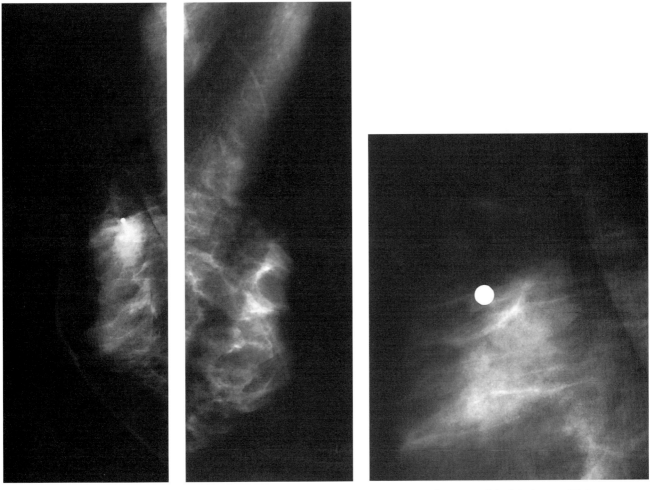

A,B   C

FIGURE 11-21. (A) Right breast, MLO view. A metallic BB marks the area of concern. **(B)** Right breast, MLO view, screen-film study, 1 year prior. **(C)** Right breast, MLO magnification view, digital. **(D)** Ultrasound image of the mass (marked by cursers). **(E)** The tumor is arranged in solid sheets and nests (H&E, 40×).

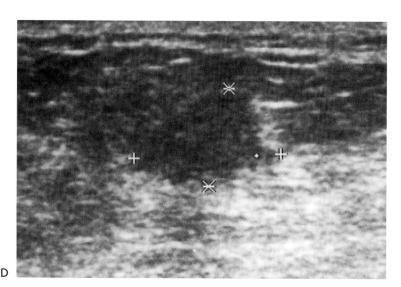

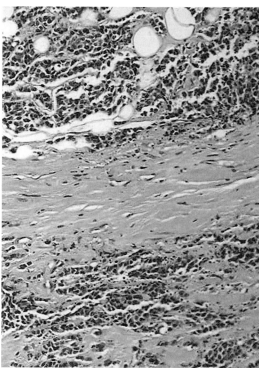

D

E

Findings

A 1.5-cm, oval, predominately circumscribed mass is present superiorly. The mass is high in density on the standard image and isodense on the additional view. The posterior margin of the mass is ill defined. No associated features are present.

Ultrasound was performed (Fig. 11-21D). Sonographically, the mass is solid, heterogeneous, horizontally oriented, and without posterior shadowing. The margins of the mass are very irregular.

The suspicious mass was sampled under ultrasound guidance for diagnosis. The patient then underwent a salvage mastectomy.

Histology

Invasive ductal carcinoma, poorly differentiated, 2-cm (Fig. 11-21E).

Comment

Even if a mass is horizontally oriented (growing along the tissue planes) with ultrasound (as in this case), one cannot assume that the mass is benign. As with mammography, the mass should be classified by its most worrisome features, such as irregular or angulated margins (as in this case), extension into a duct, and/or posterior shadowing.

CASE 22

74-year-old female with a left breast mass and spontaneous yellow nipple discharge.

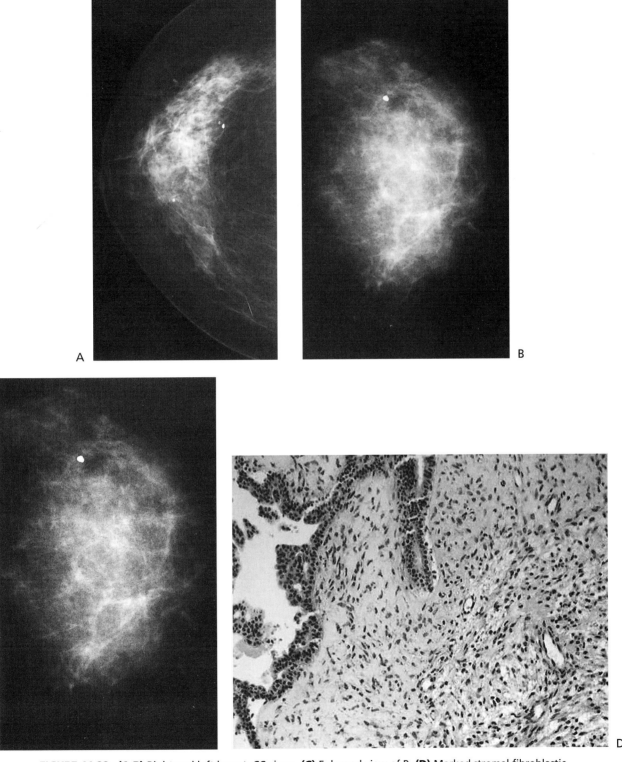

FIGURE 11-22. (A,B) Right and left breast, CC views. **(C)** Enlarged view of B. **(D)** Marked stromal fibroblastic proliferation and expansion into large "leaf-like" processes lined by hyperplastic epithelium are visualized (H&E, 100×).

Findings

The left breast is abnormal. It is smaller and denser in appearance than the right. The left breast image is grainy in appearance. The right breast is normal.

On physical examination, the left breast was replaced by a large firm mass, the skin was stretched around the mass, and yellowish fluid was leaking from the nipple. The mass was solid by ultrasound. A core biopsy was performed.

Histology

Benign phyllodes tumor (Fig. 11-22D).

The tumor was 17.2 cm in the mastectomy specimen.

No disease was identified in 3 sentinel lymph nodes.

Comment

With extremely dense breasts or breasts filled with tumor, the x-ray photons are attenuated and image quality is decreased (quantum mottle) regardless of the imaging system used.

CASE 23

68-year-old female, asymptomatic.

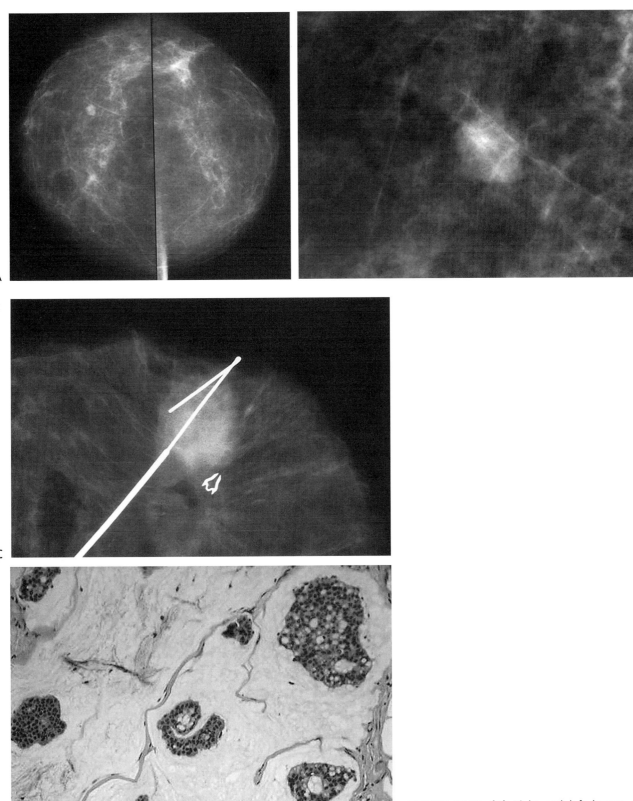

FIGURE 11-23. (A) Right and left breast, CC views, screen-film. **(B)** Right breast, CC magnification view, digital. **(C)** Specimen radiograph. **(D)** Islands of tumor are present floating in pools of extracellular mucin (H&E, 100×).

Findings

A 1-cm mass is present in the central right breast. The magnification view demonstrates the isodense mass to be irregular and ill-defined. The mass was not seen sonographically.

A core biopsy of the suspicious mass was performed to obtain a diagnosis prior to lumpectomy (Fig. 11-23C).

The mass involves the margin of the surgical specimen radiograph (Fig. 11-23C). The surgeon was notified and additional tissue was removed. Note the metallic marker clip from the previous stereotactic core biopsy.

Histology

Mucinous carcinoma, 0.8-cm (Fig. 11-23D).

Comment

Pure mucinous cancers usually have a good prognosis because of their slow growth rate and low rate of metastasis. They usually occur in older women.

CASE 24

78-year-old female, research screening study.

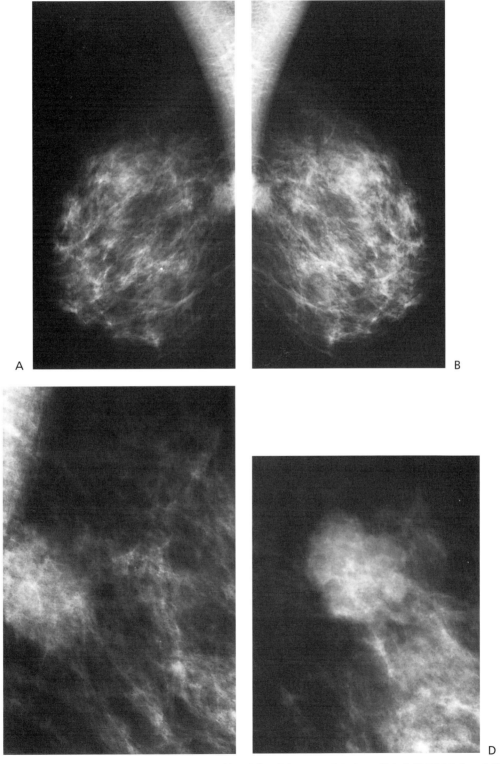

FIGURE 11-24. (A) Left breast, MLO view, screen-film. **(B)** Left breast, MLO view, digital. **(C,D)** MLO and CC magnification views, digital. **(E)** Ultrasound of the mass.

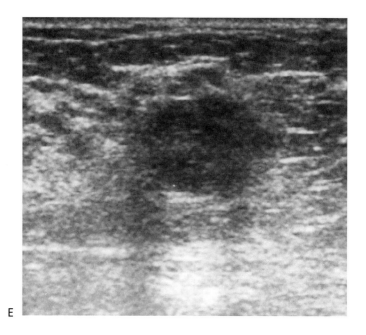

E

Findings

A 3-cm, irregular density is present in the posterior central aspect of the breast at the level of the pectoralis muscle on the MLO views. The magnification views demonstrate the margins of the mass to be indistinct and obscured on the MLO view and to be macro- and microlobulated on the CC view. No associated features are seen. The suspicious mass is seen sonographically (Fig. 11-24E).

An ultrasound guided core biopsy was performed for diagnosis.

The patient went on to have a simple mastectomy with sentinel lymph node sampling.

Histology

Invasive ductal carcinoma, poorly differentiated, 2.5-cm.

No disease was seen in the sentinel lymph nodes.

Comment

The mass is easily seen in both the screen-film and digital mammographic images.

Even though the mass is oval in shape and lobulated, it should be characterized by its most worrisome features.

CASE 25

81-year-old female, asymptomatic.

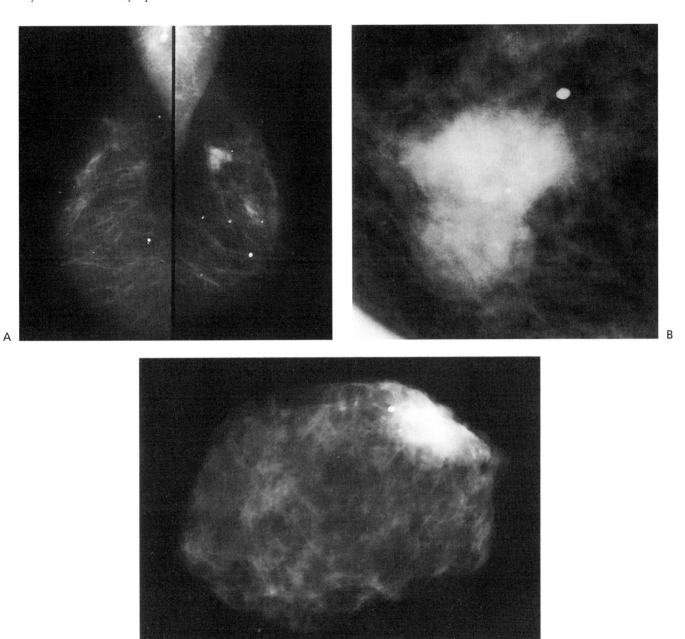

FIGURE 11-25. (A) Right and left breasts, MLO views, screen-film. **(B)** Left breast, MLO magnification view, digital. **(C)** Specimen radiograph.

Findings

A 3-cm, irregular, ill-defined, high-density mass with associated calcifications is present in the superior left breast.

An ultrasound core biopsy of the suspicious mass was performed for diagnosis prior to lumpectomy. The specimen radiograph shows the tumor to extend to a margin (Fig. 11-25C). The surgeon removed more tissue at that location.

Histology

Mucinous carcinoma, 2-cm.

The sentinel lymph node was negative for metastatic disease.

Comment

It is very important to communicate to the surgeon the findings of the specimen radiograph while the patient is still in the operating room. In this case, the surgeon excised more tissue along the involved margin. Microscopically, the new surgical margin was free of disease.

A team effort helps ensure complete removal of the abnormality and helps to decrease the patient's possibility of a second surgery for involved margins.

CASE 26

71-year-old female with a palpable right breast mass.

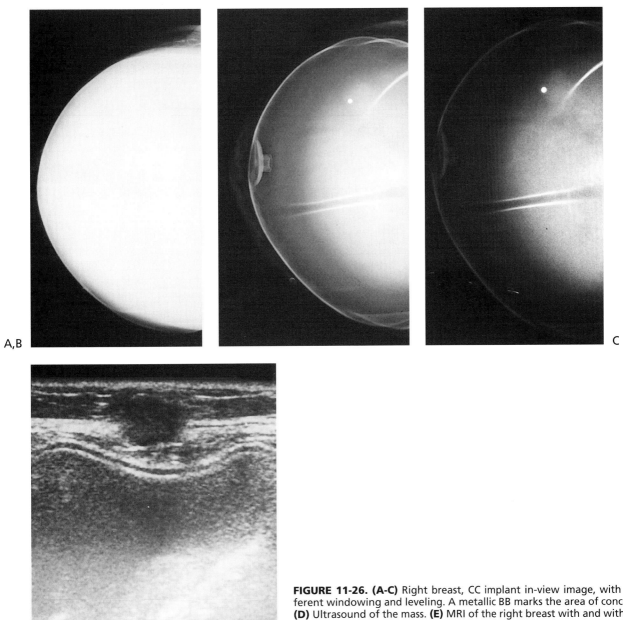

A,B

C

D

FIGURE 11-26. (A-C) Right breast, CC implant in-view image, with different windowing and leveling. A metallic BB marks the area of concern. **(D)** Ultrasound of the mass. **(E)** MRI of the right breast with and without contrast administration (3D-FLASH, T1-weighted, fat suppressed, sagittal images).

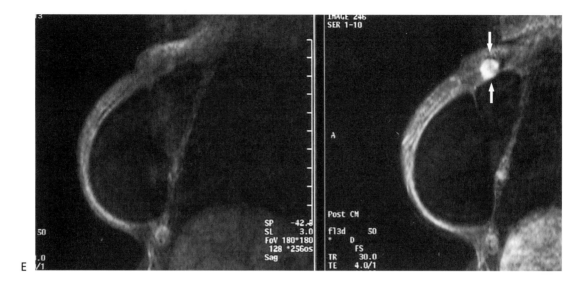

Findings

The patient has a subglandular saline implant. The first image demonstrates the implant. The metallic marker is not even seen on this image. The next image shows the marker, but it is in Figure 11-26C that a 2-cm, irregular mass is seen superiorly.

The patient was radiation phobic and would not allow additional magnification views. An ultrasound was performed and demonstrates a 2-cm suspicious mass superiorly to the implant.

To evaluate for extent of disease, breast MRI was done. On the post-contrast image, an irregular mass with predominantly peripheral enhancement (*arrows*) is present. No other foci of disease were seen. The suspicious mass was removed surgically.

Histology

Invasive ductal carcinoma, well differentiated, 1.5-cm.

Two sentinel lymph nodes were negative for tumor.

Comment

This case demonstrates the utility of digital mammography, with the use of the softcopy display system to window and level to look for abnormalities. With screen-film mammography, after the film has been exposed and processed, "what you see is what you get." The screen-film image may need to be repeated using different techniques to get good quality visualization of a mass superimposed by an implant, as in this case. This would increase the radiation dose to the patient.

CASE 27

35-year-old female with a palpable subareolar right breast mass.

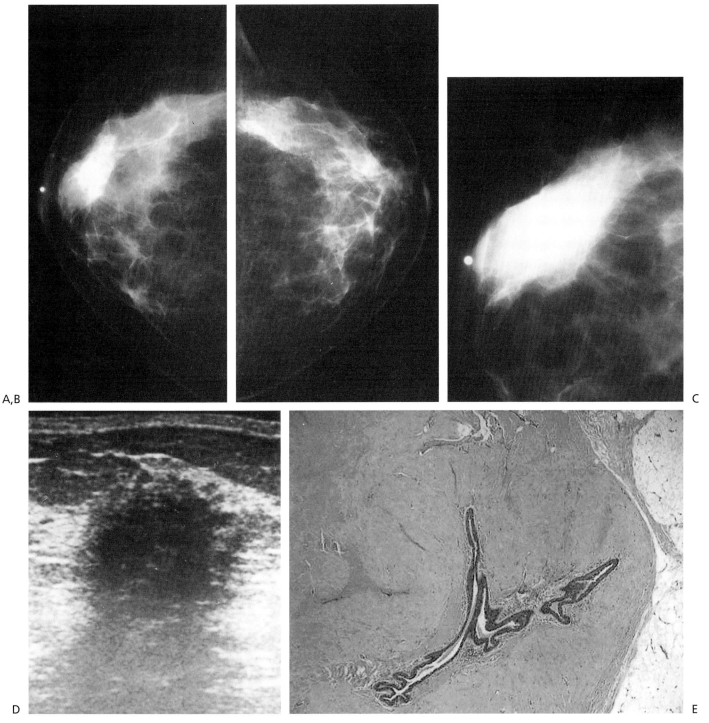

A,B

C

D

E

FIGURE 11-27. (A,B) Right and left breast, CC views. A metallic BB marks the area of concern. **(C)** Right breast, CC magnification view. **(D)** Ultrasound of the mass. **(E)** Dense stromal fibrosis with a few slightly ectatic ducts with periductal chronic inflammation is present (H&E, 20×).

Findings

A 4 to 5-cm, oval, high-density spiculated mass is present in the subareolar region of the right breast.

On physical examination, this mass was firm and measured 6 cm × 4 cm.

An ultrasound was performed. The mass is solid, hypoechoic, vertically oriented with irregular margins, and has some posterior shadowing.

Dense stromal fibrosis was diagnosed with ultrasound guided core biopsy. An incision biopsy was recommended because of the discordance between the suspicious imaging findings and the benign pathology.

Histology

Diabetic fibrous mastopathy (Fig. 11-27E).

Comment

Diabetic fibrous mastopathy is a rare benign condition that can produce a fibrotic mass or masses in the breast that mammographically are indistinguishable from cancer. This entity may manifest as bilateral masses. When the radiology and core biopsy findings are discordant, an incisional biopsy is needed to exclude carcinoma.

CASE 28

37-year-old female with a palpable subareolar left breast mass.

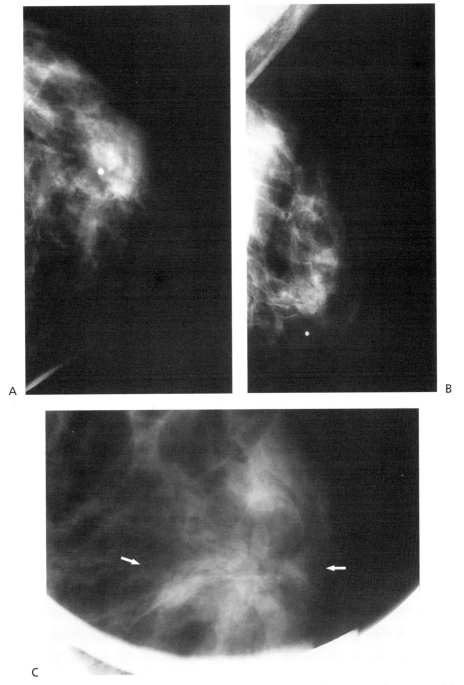

A

B

C

FIGURE 11-28. (A,B) Left breast, CC and MLO views. A metallic BB marks the area of concern. **(C)** MLO magnification view. **(D)** MLO 2nd magnification view. **(E)** CC magnification view. **(F)** 90-degree magnification view. **(G)** Specimen radiograph. **(H)** The lesion is characterized by a proliferation of epithelial elements with a central fibroelastic core (H&E, 20×).

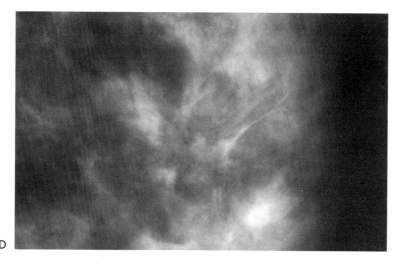

D

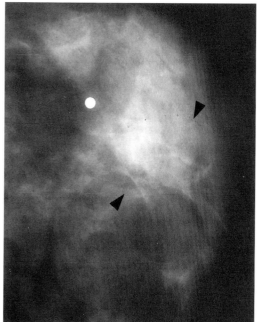

E

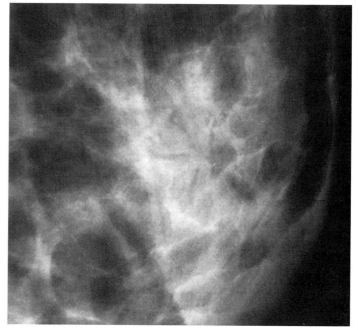

F

Findings

A 2-cm area of architectural distortion is seen beneath the metallic marker on the standard views. A possible spiculated mass (*arrows* in Fig. 11-28C) is present at the edge of the magnification paddle in the subareolar region. The MLO magnification view was repeated to center the abnormality and now only architectural distortion is identified. This is the same finding on the CC view (*arrowheads* in Fig. 11-28E).

The 90-degree magnification view shows the focal area of architectural distortion to have a lucent center and alternating lucent and opaque radiations, classic finding for a radial scar.

No mass was detected sonographically. A surgical excision was performed and the area of distortion with the alternating spiculations is visualized in the specimen (Fig. 11-28G).

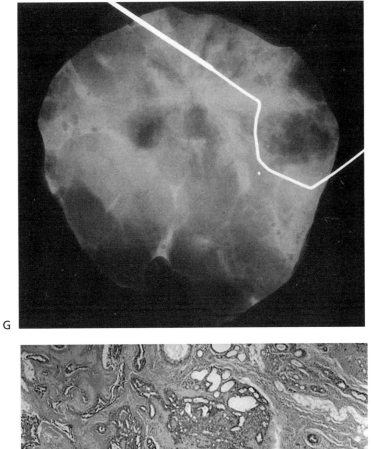

G

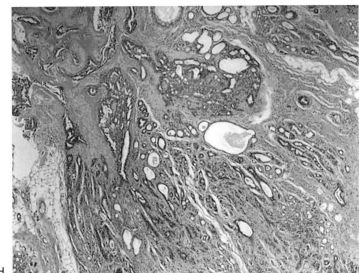

H

Histology

Radial scar (Fig. 11-28H).

Comment

A radial scar is a benign lesion characterized mammographically to have a central lucency with alternating lucent and opaque long, thin spiculations radiating from its center. Its appearance can change in different projections.

Because it can be associated with malignancy (invasive and in situ disease) complete surgical excision is recommended. Core biopsy is not recommended because there may be a sampling error, with the adjacent malignancy missed.

CASE 29

58-year-old female, 3 years status–post left lumpectomy.

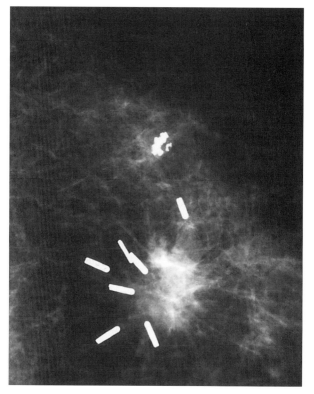

FIGURE 11-29. Left breast, CC view enlarged.

Findings

A 3-cm spiculated lesion is present in the central subareolar region of the breast. Notice the surgical clips present at the site. A low-density mass with coarse calcifications (hyalinized fibroadenoma) is present lateral to this region.

Conclusion

Postsurgical architectural distortion.

Comment

It is important to know the patient's history.

Whether from a benign biopsy or a lumpectomy, postsurgical scar should stay stable or decrease with time. If a scar increases in size and/or density, it should be considered suspicious. MRI can be helpful in this setting in distinguishing old scar from recurrent tumor in that tumor generally enhances while an old scar will usually not.

CASE 30

53-year-old female, asymptomatic.

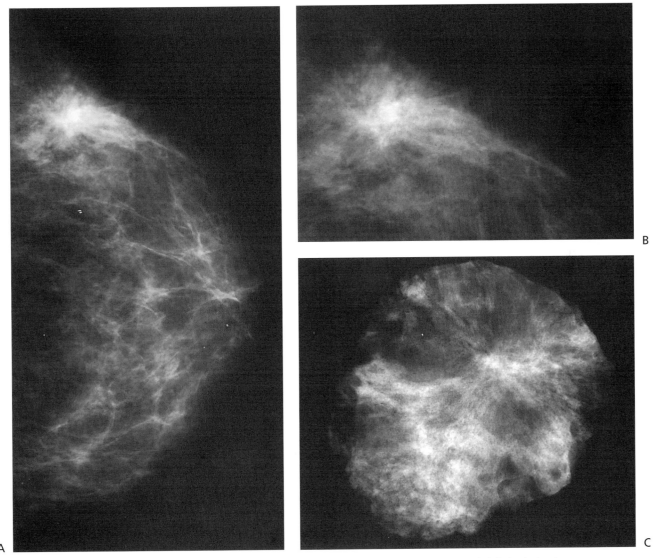

FIGURE 11-30. (A) Left breast, CC view, screen-film. **(B)** CC magnification view, digital. **(C)** The lesion is present in the specimen and its alternating lucent and opaque spiculations extend to the margins.

Findings

4-cm of architectural distortion is identified in the breast laterally.
The area was not palpable and vague shadowing was seen sonographically in one projection.

The abnormality, suspicious for a complex sclerosing lesion, was surgically removed (Fig. 11-30C).

Histology

Complex sclerosing lesion with atypia and sclerosing adenosis.
No in situ or invasive carcinoma was seen.

Comment

A complex sclerosing lesion is a radial scar that is larger than 1-cm.
Typically neither of these benign lesions are palpable nor seen sonographically.
Surgical excision is the recommended sampling method for diagnosis, as discussed previously (See Case 28).

CASE 31

52-year-old female, history of cysts.

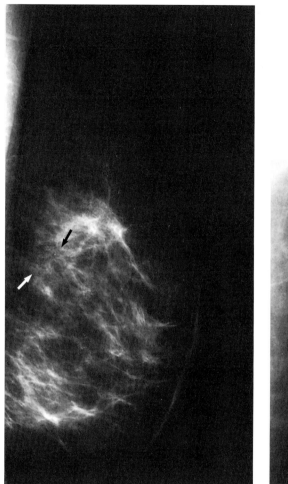
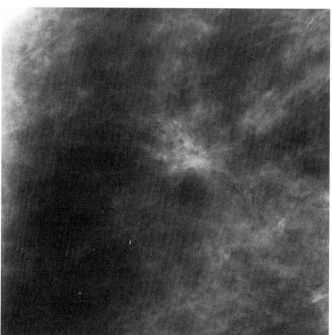

FIGURE 11-31. (A) Left breast, MLO view. **(B)** MLO magnification view.

Findings

Focal architectural distortion (*arrows*) is present in the posterior third of the breast at the level of the pectoralis muscle. Additional views confirm that it represents a spiculated mass that is highly suggestive of malignancy. The mass was sampled under ultrasound guidance prior to lumpectomy.

Histology

Invasive ductal carcinoma, well differentiated, 0.5-cm.

Comment

Additional workup of an abnormality should be performed with microfocus spot magnification views—not just spot views. Magnification views provide more information regarding an abnormality and its associated features.

CASE 32

42-year-old female with a palpable right breast mass.

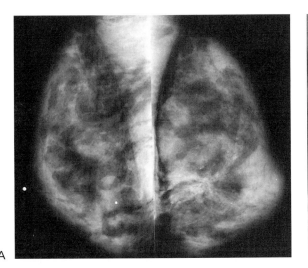

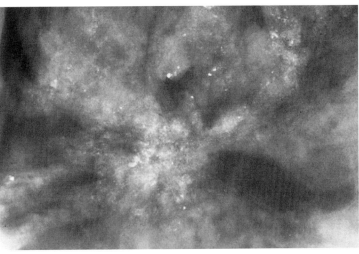

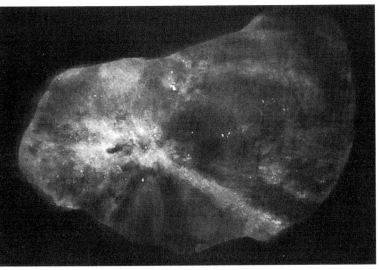

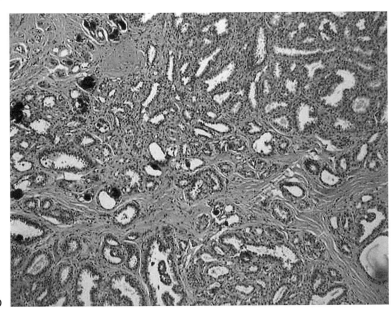

FIGURE 11-32. (A) Right and left breast, MLO views, film-screen from an outside institution. The nipples and a palpable right breast mass are marked with BBs. **(B)** Left breast, MLO magnification view, digital. **(C)** Specimen radiograph. **(D)** The calcifications are associated with benign epithelium and sclerosing adenosis (H&E 20×).

Findings

A 2-cm, oval, circumscribed isodense mass is present in the posterior central right breast.
A core biopsy of the mass was performed and yielded a diagnosis of fibroadenoma.

5-cm to 6-cm of architectural distortion is noted in the central left breast. Enumerable amorphous, round, and punctate calcifications are associated with it. The center of the distortion appears more lucent, and is suggestive of a complex sclerosing lesion. No discrete mass was appreciated on physical exam or sonographically.

Surgical excision was performed. The distortion is present along with calcifications in the specimen radiograph with involvment of the margins (Fig. 11-32C).

Histology

Complex sclerosing lesion with atypia (Fig. 11-32D).

Comment

If a radial scar or a complex sclerosing lesion is suspected, surgical excision should be performed. A core biopsy is not recommended because of the possibility of a sampling error, as these lesions can be associated with malignancy.

CASE 33

55-year-old female, history of cysts.

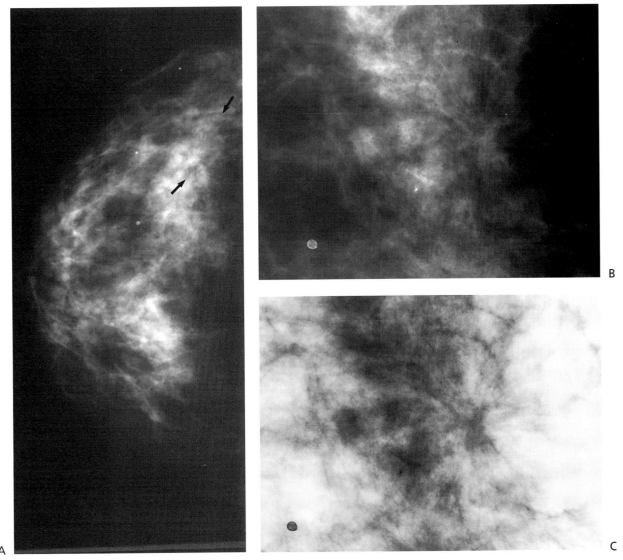

FIGURE 11-33. (A) Right breast, CC view, screen-film. **(B)** CC magnification view, digital. **(C)** Inverted image of B. **(D)** The mass with its long spiculations is present in the specimen radiograph. **(E)** Malignant epithelium with tubule formation is present (H&E, 100×).

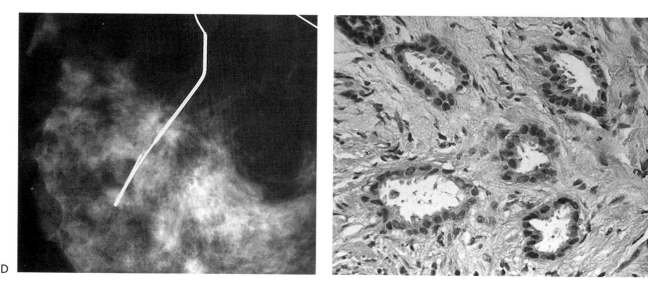

D   E

Findings

A 2-cm focal area of architectural distortion (*arrows* in Fig. 11-33A) is present in the lateral right breast. The magnification views confirm a spiculated mass without associated findings. Note the extent/length of the spiculations in the magnification view, especially in the inverted image.

The mass, highly suggestive of malignancy, was sampled with ultrasound guidance for diagnosis prior to lumpectomy (Fig. 11-33D).

Histology

Tubular carcinoma, 0.4-cm (Fig. 11-33E).

Comment

Tubular carcinoma presents as a spiculated mass. These small tumors can be multifocal or multicentric in nature so it is important to look for additional lesions. They can have bridging (sharing of spiculations) between them. Only one tumor was present in this case.

CASE 34

61-year-old female, asymptomatic.

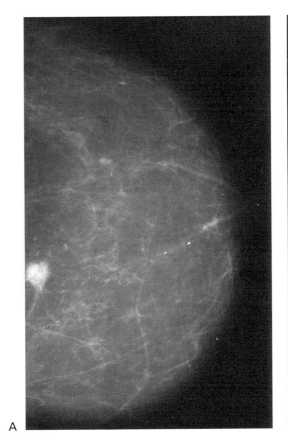

A

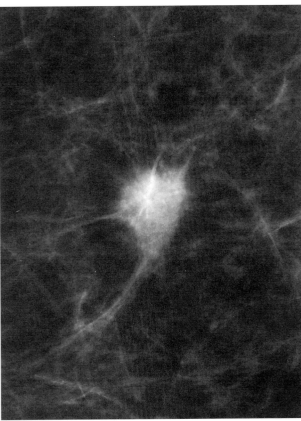

B

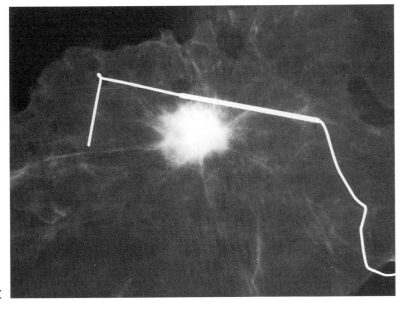

C

FIGURE 11-34. **(A)** Left breast, CC view, screen-film. **(B)** Left breast, CC magnification view, digital. **(C)** Specimen radiograph.

Findings

A 1.5-cm, spiculated, high-density mass without associated findings is present in the posterior central portion of the breast. Note the extent of the spiculations on the additional view in this fatty replaced breast. The mass, highly suggestive of malignancy, was sampled with ultrasound guidance.

The specimen radiograph from the patient's lumpectomy demonstrates the long spiculations. A few calcifications are seen adjacent to the mass (Fig. 11-34C).

Histology

Invasive ductal carcinoma, moderately differentiated, 1.3-cm, with ductal carcinoma in situ, cribriform subtype without necrosis.

Two sentinel lymph nodes were negative.

Comment

This case shows the classic mammographic appearance of an invasive breast cancer, with the mass characterized by opaque lines radiating from the margins and center of the mass.

CASE 35

73-year-old female, history of cysts.

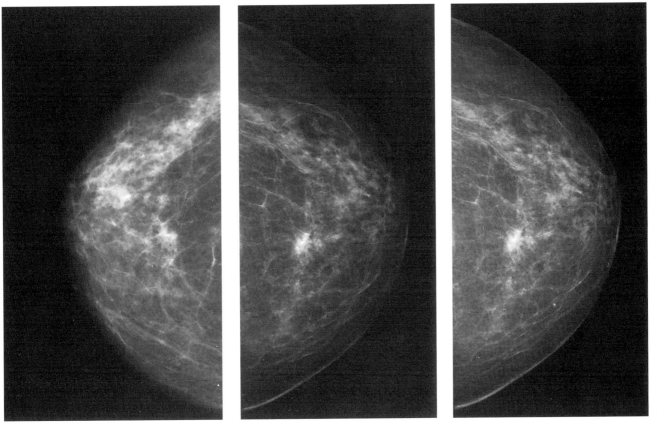

A,B   C

FIGURE 11-35. (A) Left breast, CC view, screen-film. **(B,C)** Left breast, CC views, digital with different windowing and leveling. **(D)** CC magnification view. **(E)** Specimen radiograph. **(F)** Medium sized uniform cells are arranged in the single file pattern typical of this diagnosis (H&E, 200×).

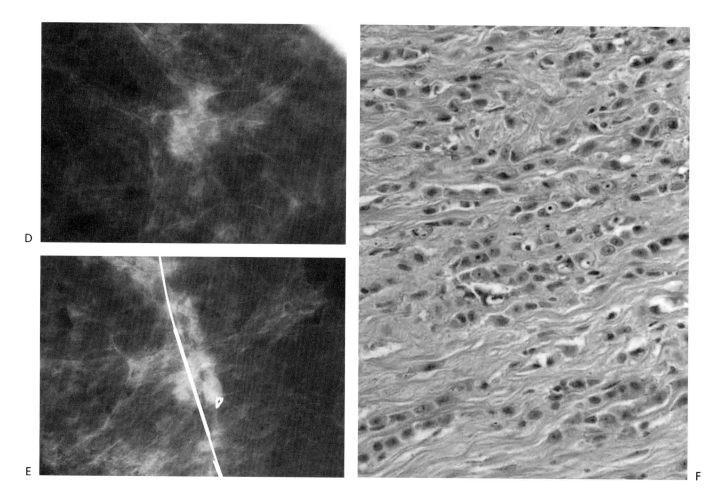

Findings

A 1.5-cm, high-density mass without associated features is present in the posterior central left breast on the digital images. The mass is isodense on the film-screen study. The margins of the mass are both spiculated and ill defined.

Since the mass, highly suggestive of malignancy, was difficult to see sonographically, a stereotactic core biopsy was performed to obtain a diagnosis. A metallic clip was placed at the site at that time. The patient then underwent a lumpectomy and the mass with its associated distortion and metallic marker clip are present in the specimen radiograph (Fig. 11-35E).

Histology

Invasive lobular carcinoma, well differentiated, 0.9-cm (Fig. 11-35F).

Comment

This case demonstrates increased conspicuity of a malignant mass with digital mammography.

CASE 36

64-year-old female, asymptomatic.

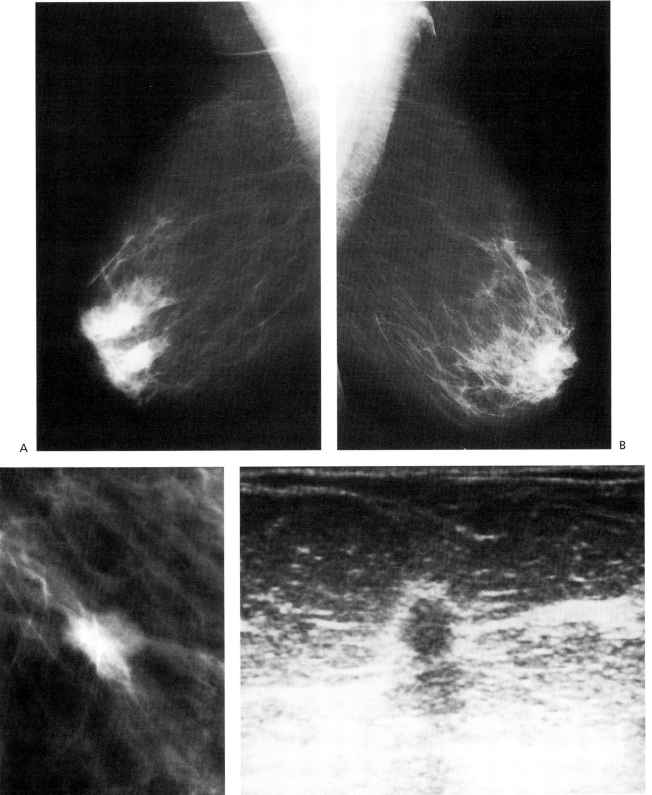

FIGURE 11-36. (A,B) Right and left breast MLO views, screen-film. **(C)** Left breast, MLO magnification view, digital. **(D)** Ultrasound of the mass.

Findings

An asymmetric density is present in the superior left breast, 8-cm from the nipple. The magnification views confirmed a 1.5-cm, spiculated, high-density mass without associated features.

Sonographically the mass is solid, hypoechoic, vertically oriented, irregular, and with some posterior shadowing. An ultrasound guided core biopsy was performed for diagnosis. The patient then underwent a lumpectomy.

Histology

Invasive ductal carcinoma, well differentiated, 1-cm.

No lymph nodes were involved.

Comment

The mass is highly suggestive of malignancy by mammography and sonography.

CASE 37

59-year-old female with a pulling sensation in the left breast.

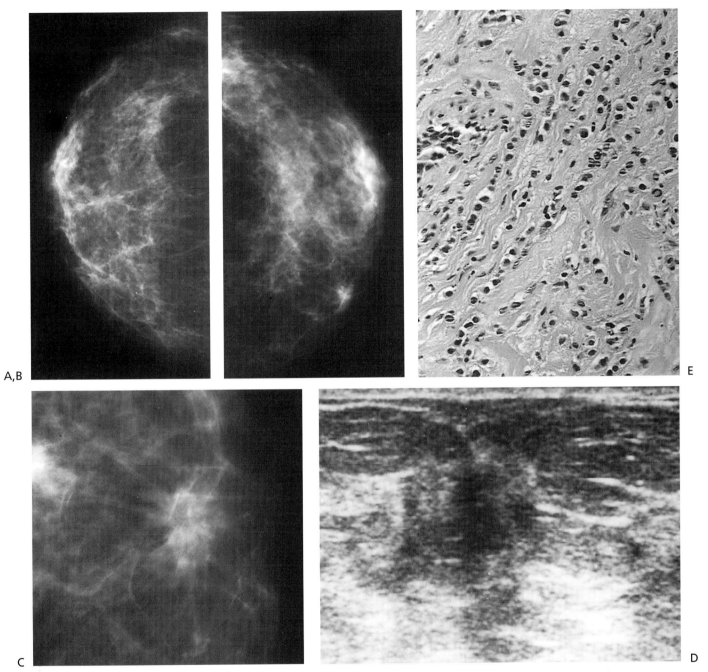

A,B

C

E

D

FIGURE 11-37. (A,B) Right and left breast, CC views. **(C)** Left breast, CC magnification view. **(D)** Ultrasound of the mass. **(E)** Small to medium sized uniform cells are arranged in single file (H&E, 200×).

Findings

A 2-cm, asymmetric density is present in the medial left breast, 6-cm from the nipple. Magnification views confirm a 2-cm, spiculated mass with associated architectural distortion.

An ultrasound of the mass demonstrates it to be solid, hypoechoic, and irregular (Fig. 11-37D). An ultrasound guided core biopsy of the mass was performed for diagnosis. The patient subsequently underwent bilateral simple mastectomies with a left sentinel node procedure.

Histology

Invasive lobular carcinoma, well differentiated, 2 cm (Fig. 11-37E).

One of five sentinel lymph nodes was positive for metastatic disease.

No tumor was identified in the right breast.

Comment

Invasive lobular carcinoma can present as a mass (spiculated or round/oval), an asymmetric density, architectural distortion, or diffuse changes of the breast. Some patients can have a normal mammogram and still have a palpable mass or thickening present. Most commonly, invasive lobular carcinoma will present as a spiculated mass, as in this case.

CASE 38

58-year-old female. Baseline mammogram.

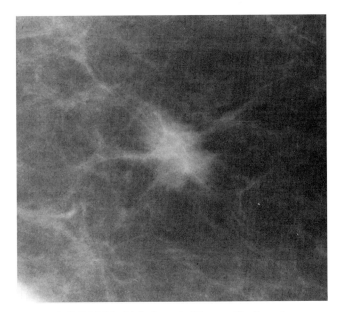

FIGURE 11-38. Right breast, CC magnification view.

Findings

A 1-cm, lobulated, isodense mass is present. Its margins are both spiculated and ill defined. No associated findings are seen. An ultrasound guided core biopsy of the mass provided the diagnosis prior to lumpectomy.

Histology

Invasive ductal carcinoma, not otherwise specified, well differentiated 1-cm.

Comment

Invasive ductal carcinoma, not otherwise specified, is the most common type of breast cancer.

CASE 39

58-year-old female, asymptomatic.

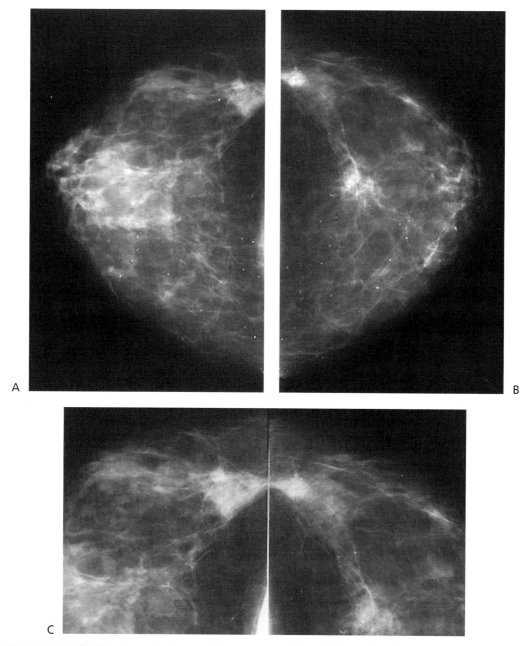

FIGURE 11-39. (A,B) Right and left breast, CC views, screen-film. **(C)** Bilateral CC views enlarged of the asymmetry of the lateral aspect of the breasts. **(D)** Left breast, CC magnification view, digital of the mass. A metallic BB was placed over a palpable mass by a technologist at the time of the additional views. **(E)** Sonography of the mass (*arrows*). **(F)** The spiculated mass is seen in the specimen radiograph. Spiculations extend to the surgical margins. The surgeon was notified and more tissue was removed at that location. **(G)** The malignant cells are uniform in size and some of the cells are in a single-file pattern (H&E, 100×).

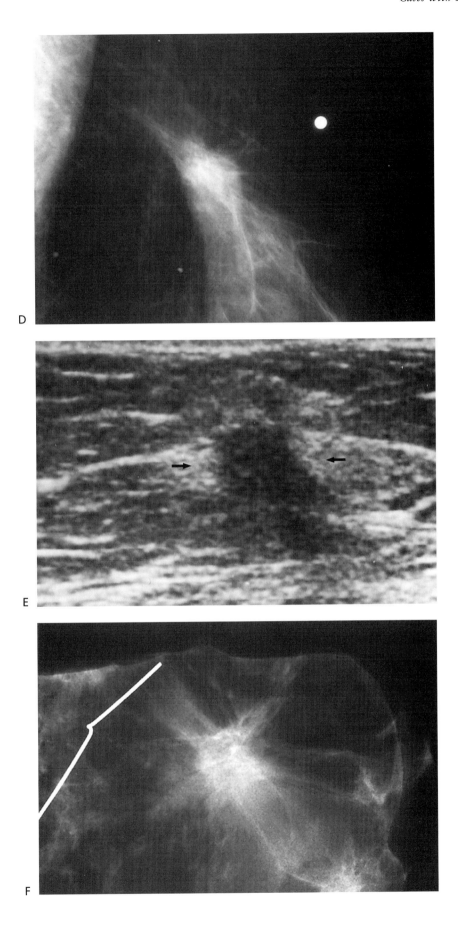

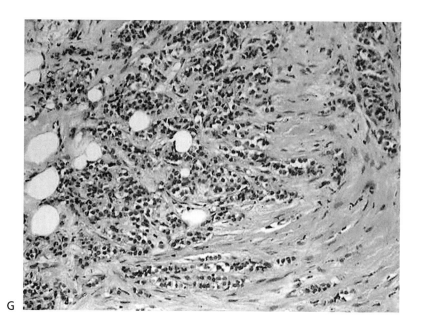

G

Findings

The patient has several areas of asymmetry involving both breasts. A subtle, 1-cm, spiculated mass is present in the lateral left breast posteriorly and is best demonstrated in the magnification view.

The mass, highly suggestive of malignancy, is easily visualized with ultrasound. An ultrasound guided core biopsy of the mass was performed to obtain a diagnosis. The patient subsequently had a lumpectomy (Fig. 11-39F).

Histology

Invasive ductal carcinoma with lobular features, moderately differentiated, 1.2-cm (Fig. 11-39G).

The sentinel lymph node was negative for disease.

Comment

It is important to evaluate all areas of the breasts. The other more obvious areas of asymmetry in both breasts represented normal tissue.

CASE 40

56-year-old female, history of cysts.

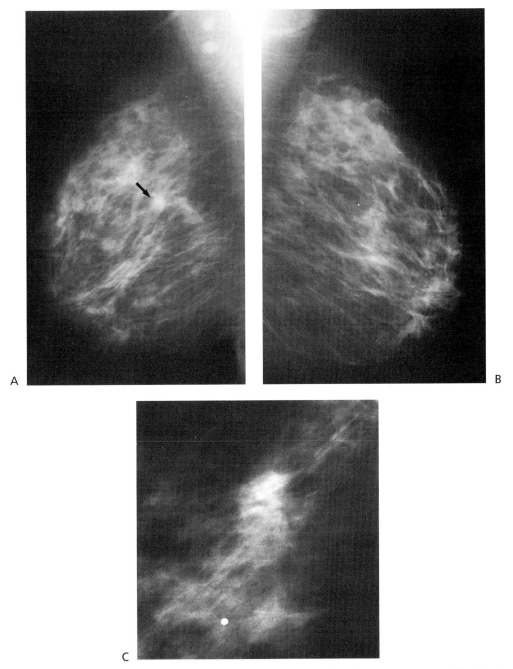

FIGURE 11-40. (A,B) Right and left breasts, MLO views screen-film. **(C)** Right breast, MLO magnification view, digital. **(D,E)** MR images of the right breast with and without contrast administration (3D FLASH, T1-weighted, fat-suppressed, sagittal images). **(F)** The lumpectomy specimen shows the spiculated mass with margin involvement.

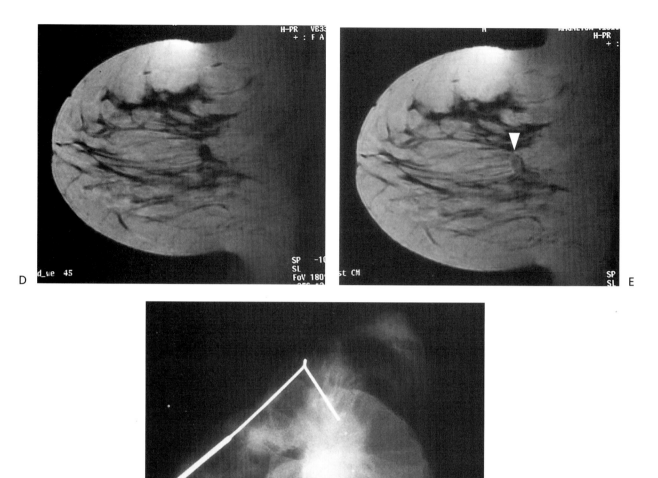

Findings

A 1.5-cm, asymmetric density with architectural distortion (*arrow* in Fig. 11-40A) is present in the right breast. This represents a spiculated, high-density mass with associated calcifications. The mass was not palpable and was poorly seen with ultrasound. Note the two abnormal right axillary lymph nodes.

The patient has a 2-cm benign appearing mass in the subareolar region of the left breast. This was a simple cyst by ultrasound.

The patient was enrolled in an MRI research study to evaluate for other foci of disease (Figs. 11-40D and 11-40E). A 1-cm enhancing, spiculated mass (*arrowhead*) is seen, and there is stronger enhancement along the periphery of the mass than centrally.

The patient then underwent a lumpectomy (Fig. 11-40F). The surgeon was notified of the findings and more tissue was taken along this margin.

Histology

Invasive ductal carcinoma, moderately differentiated, 1.2-cm. A small amount of ductal carcinoma in situ, cribriform subtype, without necrosis, was also present.

Three sentinel lymph nodes were positive for metastatic disease.

CASE 41

76-year-old female, 5 years status–post right lumpectomy and radiation therapy.

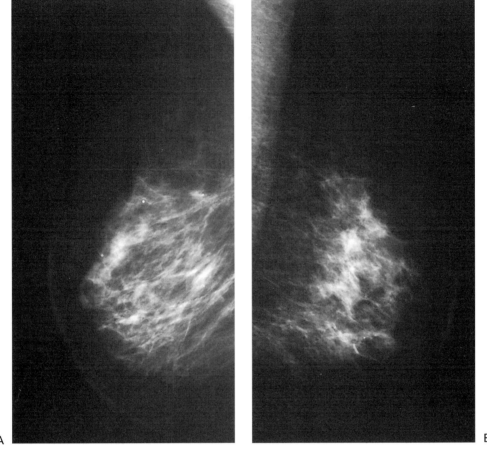

A   B

FIGURE 11-41. **(A,B)** Right and left breast, MLO views. **(C,D)** Right and left breast, CC views. **(E,F)** Left breast MLO and CC magnification views. **(G)** Left lumpectomy specimen radiograph.

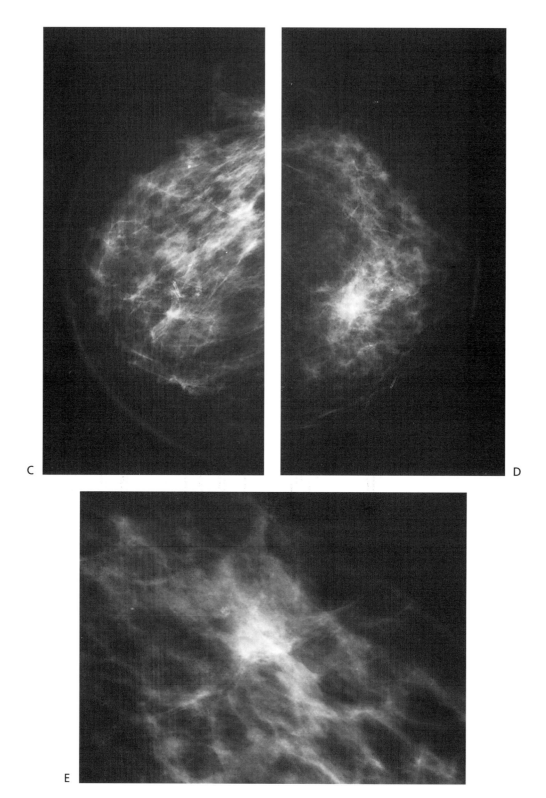

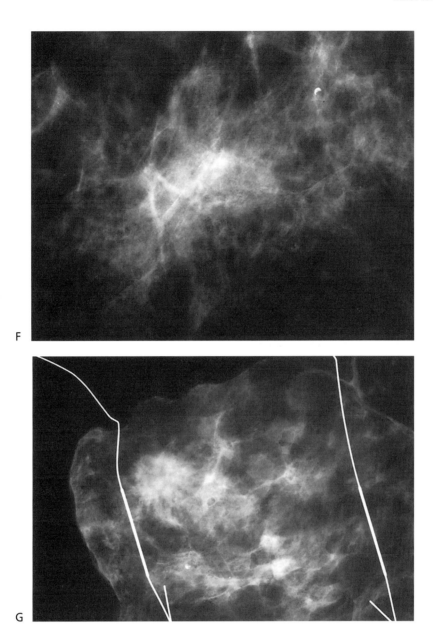

Findings

The overall density of the right breast is increased, and there is skin thickening. Distortion is seen in the upper outer quadrant of the breast. These findings are related to postsurgical and postradiation changes.

In the upper inner quadrant of the left breast, a 2-cm, asymmetric density is present. Additional views demonstrate the density to represent an ill-defined mass without associated features. This suspicious mass was sampled under ultrasound guidance. The left lumpectomy specimen radiograph (Fig. 11-41G) demonstrates the ill-defined mass to be spiculated.

Histology

Invasive ductal carcinoma, moderately differentiated, 1.5-cm, with cribriform and comedo-type ductal carcinoma in situ. No sentinel lymph nodes were involved.

Comments

This case demonstrates typical postsurgical and postradiation changes in the right breast.
It is of course always important to evaluate both breasts thoroughly.

CASE 42

60-year-old male with a palpable left breast mass.

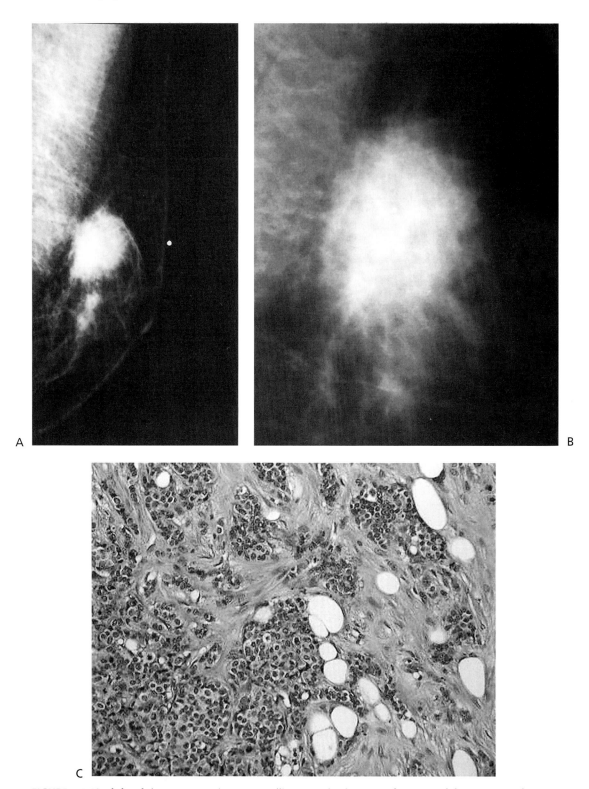

A

B

C

FIGURE 11-42. (A) Left breast, MLO view. A metallic BB marks the area of concern. **(B)** MLO magnification view. **(C)** The tumor is arranged in solid sheets and nests (H&E, 100×).

Findings

A 3-cm, spiculated, high-density mass with associated calcifications is present in the subareolar region. Inferiorly to the large mass there is a 1.5-cm, bilobed, irregular density, which was confirmed sonographically to represent a separate mass. The left breast (not shown) was normal.

Conclusion

Masses highly suggestive of malignancy in a male.

Histology

Invasive ductal carcinoma, poorly differentiated, with comedo-type ductal carcinoma in situ with necrosis.

The invasive tumors measured 3.5-cm and 1.5-cm in the mastectomy specimen (Fig. 11-42C).

One of two sentinel lymph nodes was positive for metastatic disease.

Comment

Male and female breast cancers have the same mammographic appearance.

CASE 43

57 year-old-female, asymptomatic.

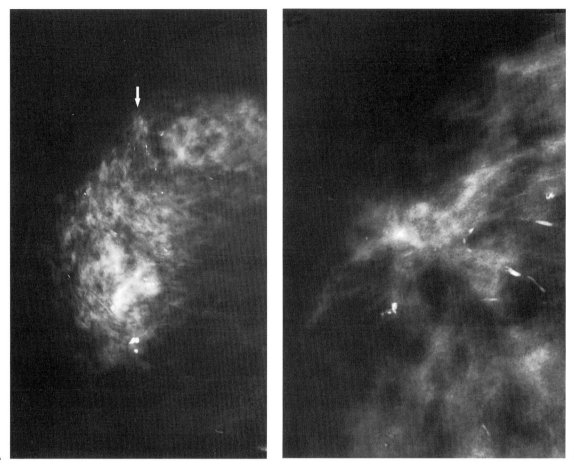

A

B

FIGURE 11-43. (A) Right breast, CC view, screen-film. **(B)** CC magnification view. **(C)** The mass with associated calcifications is easily seen in specimen radiograph.

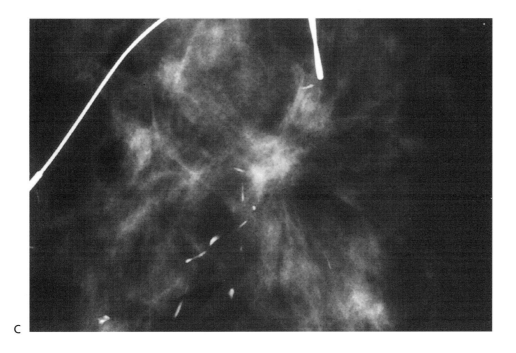

C

Findings

Two centimeters of architectural distortion is detected in the breast laterally (*arrow* in Fig. 11-43A).
Additional imaging demonstrates a spiculated mass with associated calcifications. The mass, highly suggestive of malignancy, was sampled by ultrasound guidance. The patient then underwent a lumpectomy (Fig. 11-43C).

Histology

Infiltrating ductal carcinoma, well-differentiated, 0.9-cm in size.

Ductal carcinoma in situ, cribriform subtype without necrosis, was associated with the mass. The coarse calcifications were associated with secretory disease.

Comment

The heterogeneous breast tissue obscures the extent of the spiculations of the mass even in this digital mammogram.

CASE 44

48-year-old female with a palpable right breast mass for 6 months.

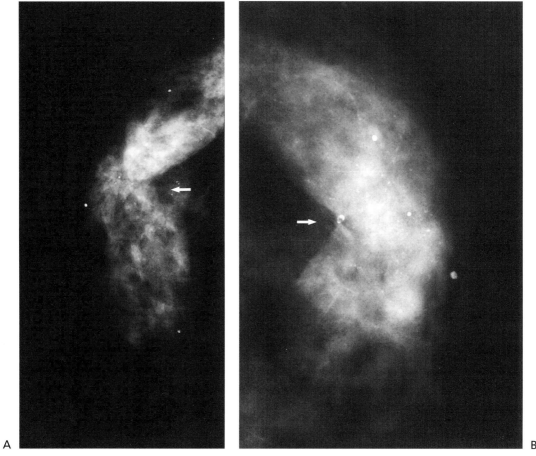

FIGURE 11-44. (A) Right breast, CC view. **(B)** CC magnification view. The images are displayed back to back.

Findings

A large subareolar mass with architectural distortion is present. Note the parenchymal retraction (*arrow*) in the breast. The associated pleomorphic calcifications are best seen in the magnification view. A core biopsy was performed.

Histology

Invasive ductal carcinoma, poorly differentiated, with extensive comedo-type ductal carcinoma in situ with necrosis.

The patient had little response to neoadjuvant chemotherapy prior to her mastectomy. The tumor was 3.5-cm, with extensive intraductal carcinoma. The patient also had metastatic involvement of one of three sentinel lymph nodes.

Comment

This is an example of a "tent sign"–parenchymal retraction of the posterior border of the glandular tissue. Straight lines in the breast should be viewed with suspicion. If there is no history of previous surgery, then a malignant process should be assumed and sought.

CASE 45

71-year-old female with a physician-detected right breast mass medially.

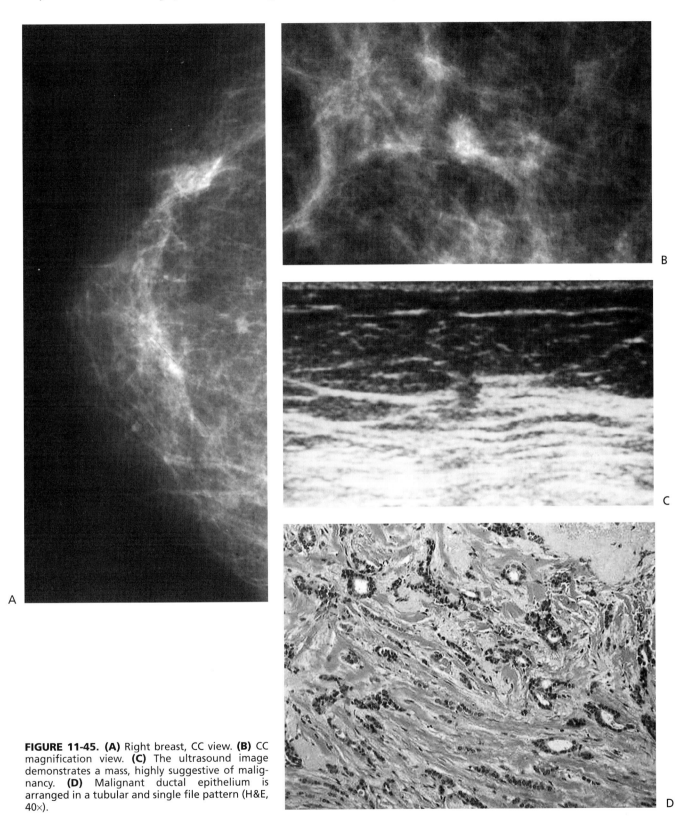

A

B

C

D

FIGURE 11-45. (A) Right breast, CC view. **(B)** CC magnification view. **(C)** The ultrasound image demonstrates a mass, highly suggestive of malignancy. **(D)** Malignant ductal epithelium is arranged in a tubular and single file pattern (H&E, 40×).

Findings

A less than 1-cm mass is identified in the retroglandular fat at the level of the nipple line. Additional imaging confirms a spiculated mass with associated calcifications.

The ultrasound image demonstrates a less than 1-cm, solid, hypoechoic, vertically oriented mass without posterior shadowing. The mass is not palpable. An ultrasound guided core biopsy of the mass was performed for diagnosis. The patient then underwent a lumpectomy.

Histology

Invasive ductal carcinoma with lobular features, well differentiated, 0.4-cm, associated with cribriform-type ductal carcinoma in situ without necrosis (Fig. 11-45D). Calcifications were associated with the in situ disease.

Two sentinel lymph nodes were negative for metastatic disease.

Comment

Remember to evaluate the entire breast and not focus just on the history. The area of physician-detected mass concerned medially represented normal fat lobules.

CASE 46

46-year-old female, history of cysts.

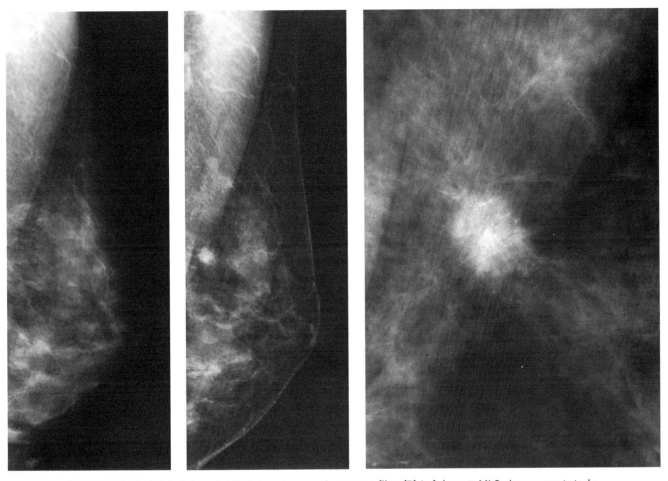

A,B   C

FIGURE 11-46. (A) Left breast, MLO view, 1-year prior, screen-film. **(B)** Left breast, MLO view, current study, digital. **(C)** MLO magnification view, digital.

Findings

In the interval, a 1-cm, spiculated, high-density mass with associated calcifications has developed posteriorly at the level of the pectoralis muscle. The nonpalpable mass, highly suggestive of malignancy, was sampled under ultrasound guidance prior to breast conservation surgery.

Histology

Invasive ductal carcinoma, well differentiated, 1.2-cm, with adjacent comedo and cribriform ductal carcinoma in situ.

Two sentinel lymph nodes were negative for tumor involvement.

Comment

A mammogram is recommended every year after the age of 40.

CASE 47

75-year-old female with history of benign biopsies.

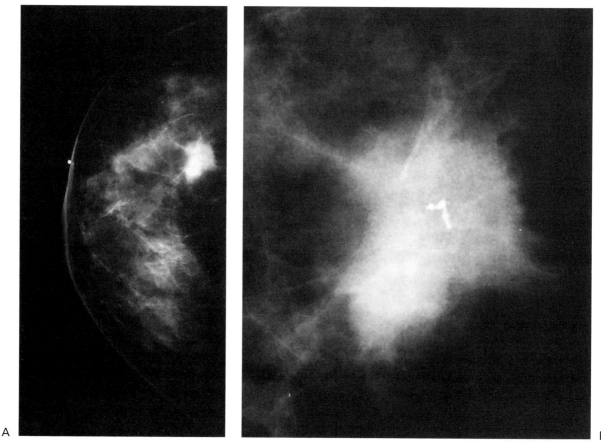

FIGURE 11-47. (A) Right breast, CC view. A skin lesion is marked with a metallic marker. **(B)** CC magnification view.

Findings

A 2.5-cm, irregular, spiculated, high-density mass with associated calcifications is identified in the posterior aspect of the breast just lateral to the nipple line. The spiculated margins and its associated calcifications are best appreciated on the magnification view.

Histology

Invasive ductal carcinoma, poorly differentiated, 2.1-cm, with comedo-type ductal carcinoma in situ.

One of three sentinel lymph nodes was involved with tumor.

Comment

The calcifications in the mass appear coarse. These calcifications are comedo-type ductal carcinoma and should not be confused with benign-type calcifications. When calcifications such as these are observed without a mass, comedo-type ductal carcinoma in situ should be considered.

CASE 48

39-year-old female with a palpable right breast mass.

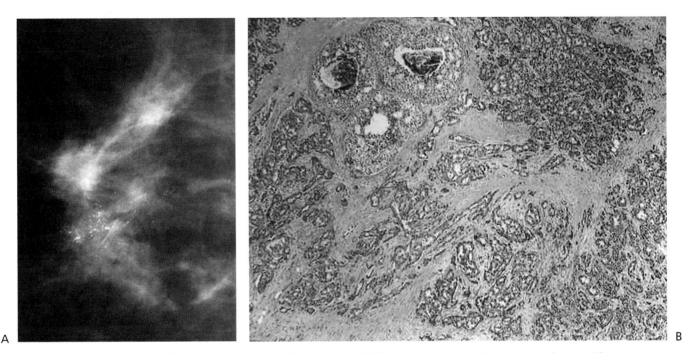

A

B

FIGURE 11-48. (A) Right breast, CC magnification view. **(B)** The tumor is arranged in tubules and nests with ductal carcinoma in situ—upper left (H&E, 40×).

Findings

A 1-cm, spiculated, high-density mass with adjacent 3-cm of ductally oriented pleomorphic and linear (casting type) calcifications are seen in the image.

An ultrasound guided core biopsy of the mass, highly suggestive of malignancy, confirmed the diagnosis of invasive carcinoma. The patient then underwent bilateral simple mastectomies.

Histology

Invasive ductal carcinoma, moderately differentiated, 1.2-cm, with adjacent 8-cm of ductal carcinoma in situ, comedo and cribriform type with necrosis (Fig. 11-48B).

One of three sentinel lymph nodes was positive for metastatic involvement.

Comment

The majority of the patient's ductal carcinoma in situ was mammographically and clinically occult disease.

CASE 49

35-year-old, postpartum, lactating patient with a palpable right breast mass.

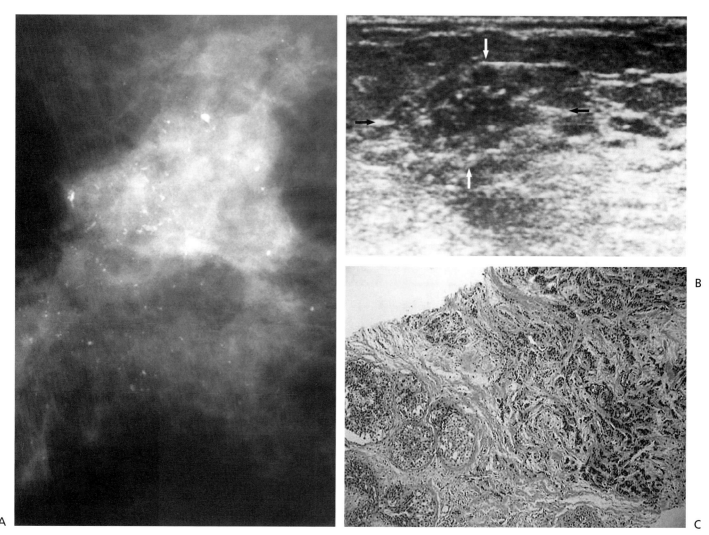

A

B

C

FIGURE 11-49. (A) Right CC magnification view of the area of concern. **(B)** Ultrasound of the palpable mass. **(C)** Malignant epithelium is arranged in sheets and nests with adjacent ductal carcinoma in situ–lower left (H&E, 20×).

Findings

Lactational changes are present. Extensive pleomorphic calcifications are seen with a 3-cm density.

Ultrasound demonstrates a 2.5-cm mass (*arrows* Fig. 11-49B). The mass is solid, heterogeneous with echogenic foci (calcifications) irregular, and horizontally oriented. A core biopsy of the suspicious mass was performed under ultrasound guidance.

Histology

Invasive ductal carcinoma, poorly differentiated, with solid and comedo-type ductal carcinoma in situ, with and without necrosis (Fig. 11-49C).

Comment

The patient underwent neoadjuvant chemotherapy followed by a mastectomy.

No invasive or in situ disease was found in the mastectomy specimen, and calcifications were associated with fibrocystic changes.

CASE 50

64-year-old female with a palpable left breast mass.

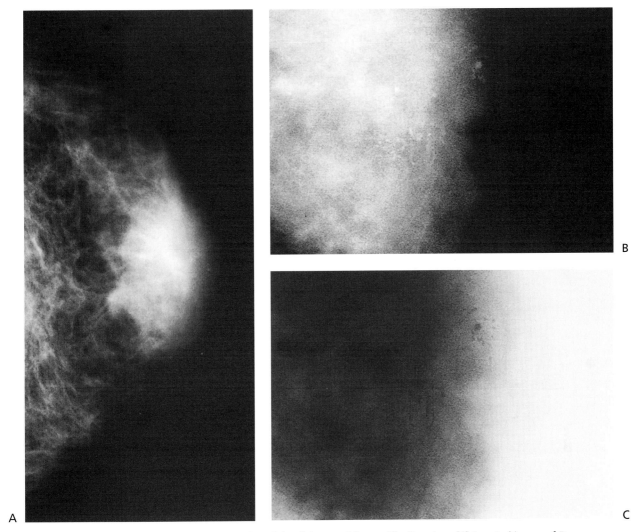

FIGURE 11-50. (A) Left breast, CC view. **(B)** Left breast, CC magnification view. **(C)** Inverted image of **B**.

Findings

The left breast is abnormal. A 7-cm × 5-cm mass with associated calcifications is present in the subareolar region. The associated pleomorphic calcifications are difficult to see on the magnification view, even in the inverted mode. The image is grainy. The trabecular markings are thickened. Edematous changes are noted.

The patient's skin was erythematous, edematous, and ulcerated. A core biopsy of the palpable mass was performed for diagnosis.

Conclusion

Inflammatory breast carcinoma.

Histology

Infiltrating ductal carcinoma, poorly differentiated, with comedo-type ductal carcinoma in situ, with necrosis.

Comment

Even with digital mammography, if the breast is extremely dense or unable to be compressed (secondary to diffuse tumor), the image can be degradated secondary to quantum mottle.

12

DIGITAL MAMMOGRAPHY CASES WITH CALCIFICATIONS

CHERIE M. KUZMIAK

CASE 1

82-year-old female with a palpable right breast mass.

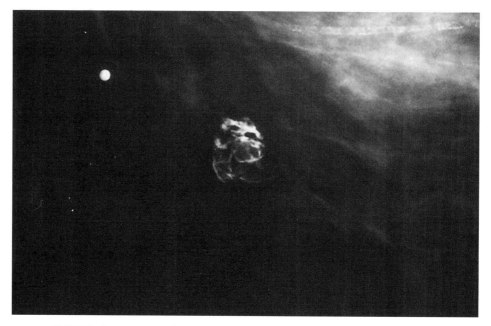

FIGURE 12-1. CC magnification view. A metallic BB marks the area of concern.

Findings
A 1-cm, lucent mass with peripheral (eggshell type) calcification is present.

Conclusion
Calcified oil cyst/fat necrosis.

Comment
Calcifications that have a lucent center are benign.

CASE 2

32-year-old female, research screening study.

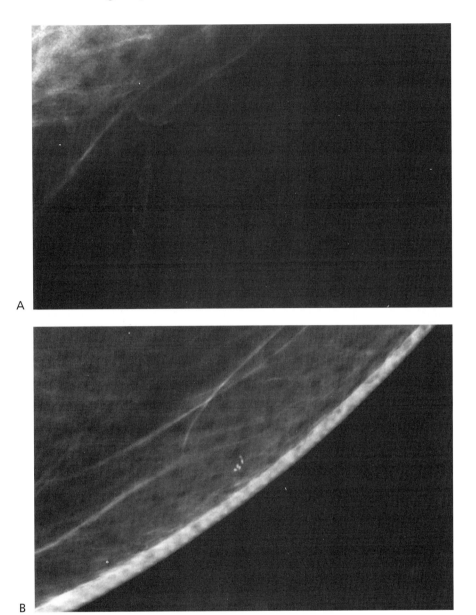

FIGURE 12-2. (A) Left breast, CC view enlarged, screen-film. **(B)** Left breast, CC view enlarged, digital.

Findings

No definite finding is visulized on the screen-film study.
On the digital study, a cluster of oval calcifications is seen.

Conclusion

Benign calcifications, lobular type.

Comment

This is a case where the finding is not seen on the screen-film study because it is in the subcutaneous tissue. It could only be seen by "hot lighting" the image.

CASE 3

62-year-old female, asymptomatic.

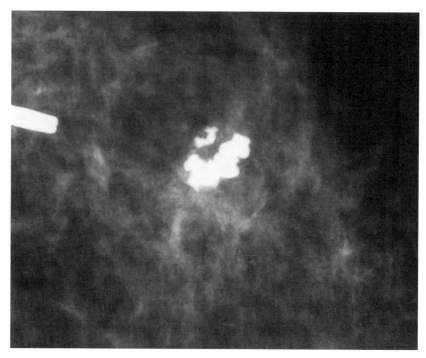

FIGURE 12-3. Left breast, CC view enlarged.

Findings

High-density, coarse "popcorn type" calcifications are seen in a low-density mass. Note the surgical clip posterior to it.

Conclusion

Hyalinized fibroadenoma.

Comment

This is a classic mammographic appearance for a fibroadenoma.

CASE 4

57-year-old female, history of implants.

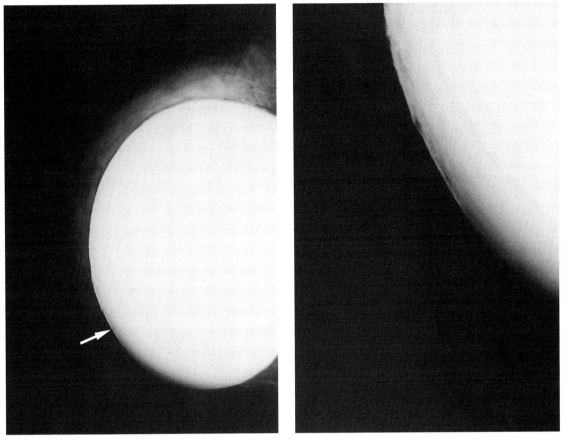

A   B

FIGURE 12-4. (A) Right breast, CC implant in-view image. **(B)** CC view enlarged.

Findings

The patient has a subglandular silicone implant with irregularity of the capsule anteriorly (*arrow*) in Figure 12-4A. The irregularity represents calcifications on the surface of the implant, and not silicon from a ruptured implant.

Conclusion

Capsular calcifications.

Comment

Capsular calcifications are a common finding.

CASE 5

58-year-old female, asymptomatic.

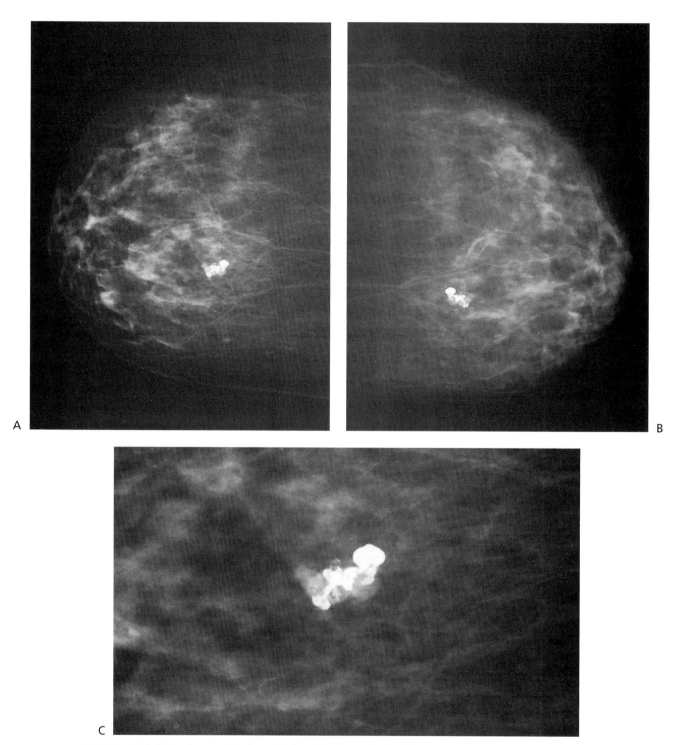

FIGURE 12-5. Right breast CC views displayed back to back. **(A)** Digital. **(B)** Screen-film. **(C)** CC view enlarged, digital.

Findings

A 1.5-cm, lobulated, low-density mass with coarse calcifications is seen in the posterior central portion of the breast.

Conclusion

Hyalinized fibroadenoma.

Comment

The benign mass is seen well with both digital and screen-film mammography.

CASE 6

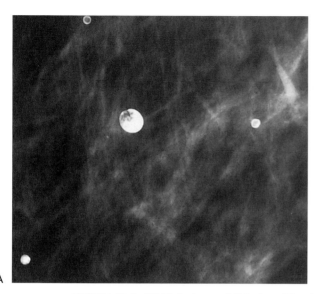 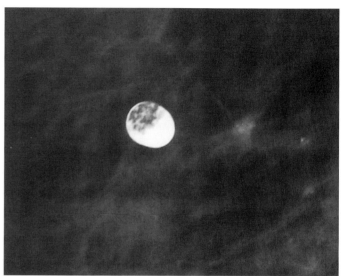

FIGURE 12-6. (A) Right breast, MLO view. **(B)** Enlarged view of **A**.

Findings

Calcifications with lucent centers.

Conclusion

Calcified oil cysts.

Comment

These are so-called "eggshell type" calcifications.

CASE 7

Two different patients.

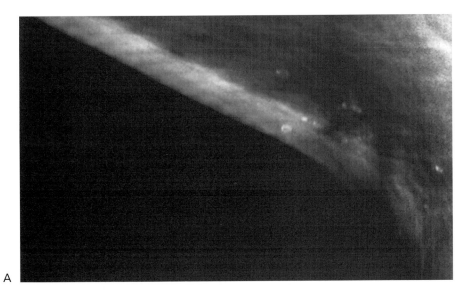

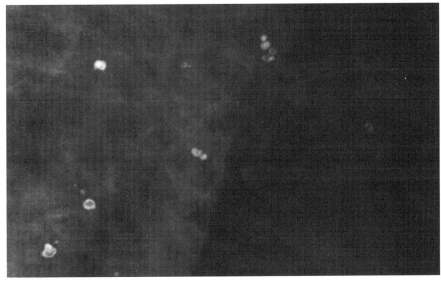

FIGURE 12-7. (A) Right breast, CC view enlarged. **(B)** Left breast, MLO view enlarged.

Findings

Tiny round to oval calcifications with lucent centers are seen. The calcifications are present in the skin.

Conclusion

This is the classic appearance of dermal calcifications.

CASE 8

78-year-old female, 1 year status–post right lumpectomy.

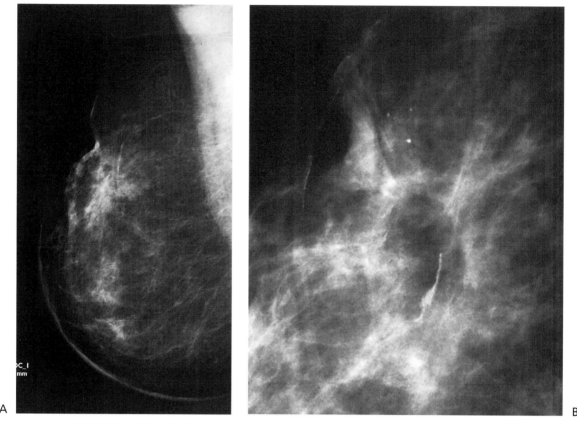

FIGURE 12-8. (A) Right breast, MLO view. **(B)** MLO magnification view of lumpectomy site.

Findings

Architectural distortion with skin thickening is noted in the superior portion of the breast. A 2-cm, oval, lucent mass with calcifications along its margins is seen at the lumpectomy site.

Conclusion

Fat necrosis.

Comment

It is recommended that standard views of the breasts and microfocus spot magnification views of the lumpectomy site be obtained for breast conservation patients to help evaluate for recurrent disease. Statistically, most ipsilateral recurrences are at the lumpectomy site or adjacent to it.

CASE 9

42-year-old female, history of cysts.

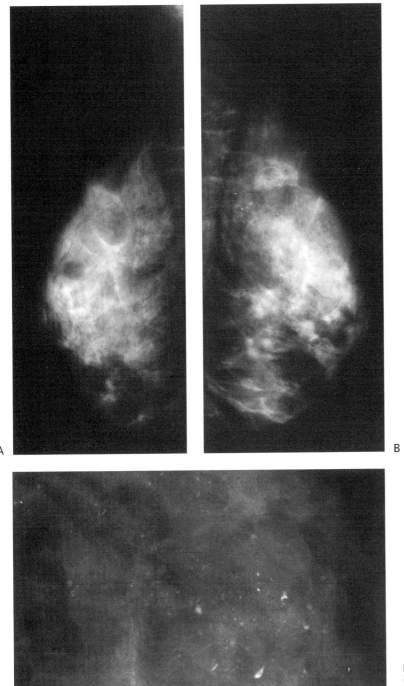

A

B

C

FIGURE 12-9. **(A,B)** Right and left breast, MLO views. **(C)** Left breast, CC magnification view. **(D)** Left breast, 90-degree magnification view.

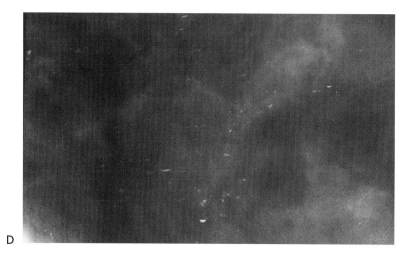

D

Findings

Calcifications are present in the superior left breast. The CC magnification view shows the majority of the calcifications to be round and "smudgy" in appearance. The 90-degree magnification view demonstrates the calcium to change shape with the different projection. Now the calcifications are crescentic in shape, so-called "tea cupping."

Conclusion

Benign findings, diagnostic of milk of calcium.

Comment

When evaluating calcifications, a microfocus spot magnification view in the CC and 90-degree projections should be obtained. If there is not enough sediment in the microcysts, the crescentic layering may not be seen on the MLO view.

CASE 10

57-year-old female, asymptomatic.

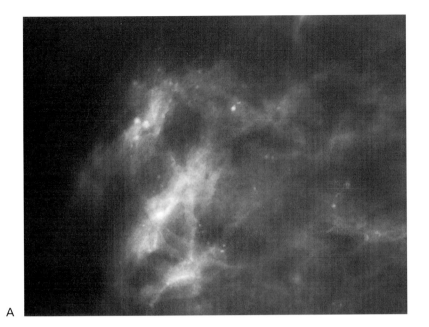

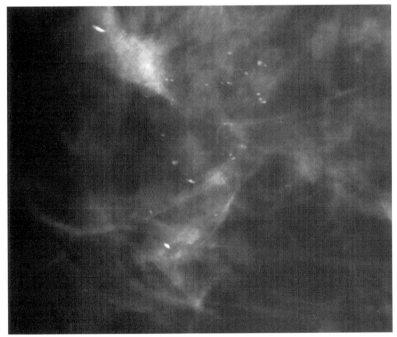

FIGURE 12-10. (A) Right breast, CC magnification view. **(B)** Right breast, 90-degree magnification view.

Findings

The calcifications change shape in the different projections.

Conclusion

This is another demonstration of milk of calcium.

CASE 11

Three different patients.

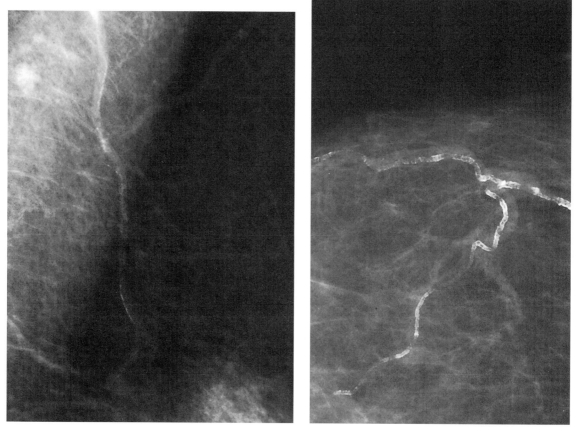

FIGURE 12-11. (A–C) MLO, CC, and CC views enlarged.

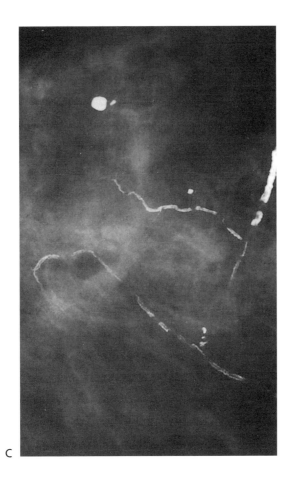

C

Findings

Parallel "train-track type" calcifications are visualized along a low-density tubular structure.

Conclusion

Vascular calcifications.

Comment

Sometimes it is difficult to tell if calcifications are vascular, especially if the calcifications are seen only along one side of the vessel or if the vessel is not well seen. Magnification views can be helpful in these situations.

CASE 12

58-year-old female, asymptomatic.

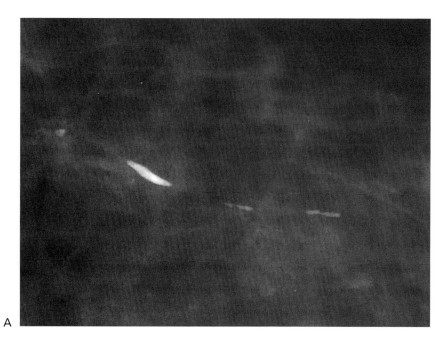

A

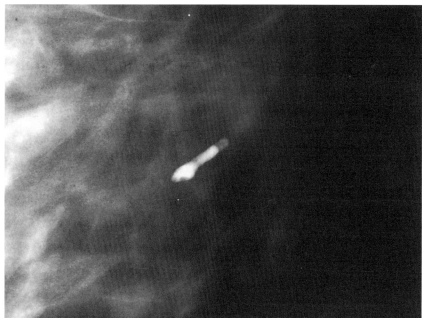

B

FIGURE 12-12. (A,B) Left breast, MLO view enlarged.

Findings

Coarse, rod-like calcifications with ductal orientation.

Conclusion

Secretory calcifications.

Comment

Sometimes these macrocalcifications will have a lucent center.

CASE 13

52-year-old female, history of implants for 20 years.

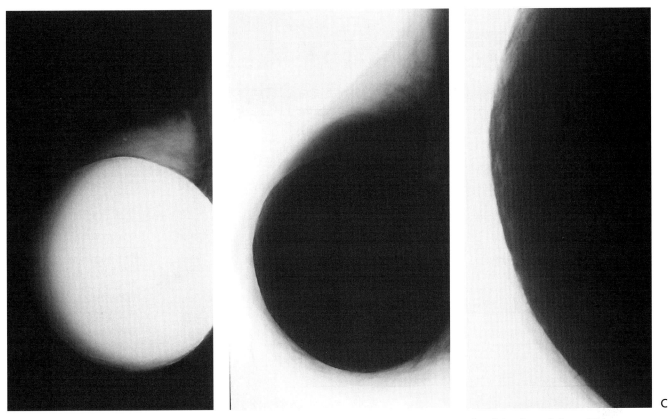

A,B   C

FIGURE 12-13. (A) Right breast, MLO implant in-view image. **(B)** Inverted view of A. **(C)** Enlarged view of B.

Findings

A subglandular silicone implant with subtle contour irregularity is seen. Calcifications are noted along the surface of the capsule. The implant is round in appearance.

Conclusion

Capsular contraction of the implant with calcifications along its surface.

Comment

It is common for implants to become more rounded in appearance because of capsular contraction and to develop capsular calcifications over time.

CASE 14

84-year-old female with a palpable right breast mass.

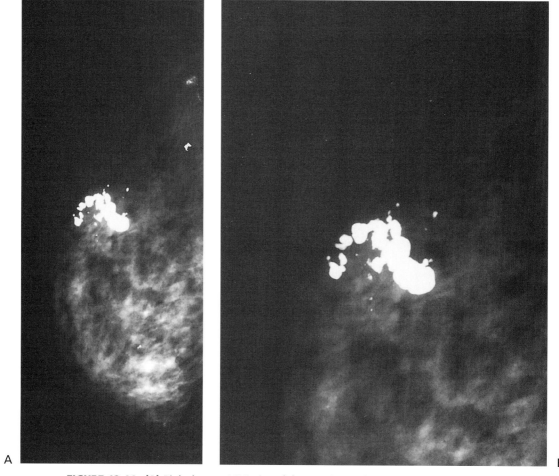

A   B

FIGURE 12-14. (A) Right breast, MLO view. **(B)** MLO view enlarged of the palpable mass.

Findings

Coarse, high-density, "popcorn type" calcifications are associated with a 3-cm, low-density mass in the superior portion of the breast. Note the smaller calcified mass near the axilla.

Conclusion

Hyalinized fibroadenomas.

Comment

Fibroadenomas are easy to diagnose when they have this classic appearance. However, they may present as a mass without calcifications or a cluster of calcifications without a mass. In these cases, additional workup may be necessary.

CASE 15

47-year-old female, asymptomatic.

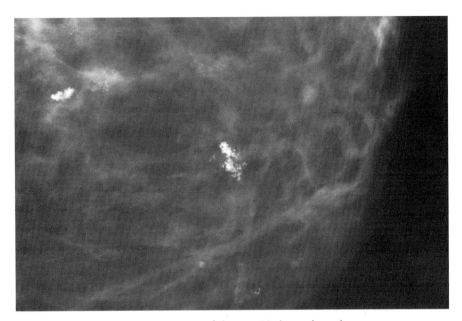

FIGURE 12-15. Left breast, CC view enlarged.

Findings

Multiple clusters of coarse calcifications are present without a discrete mass.

Conclusion

Dystrophic calcifications.

CASE 16

63-year-old female, asymptomatic.

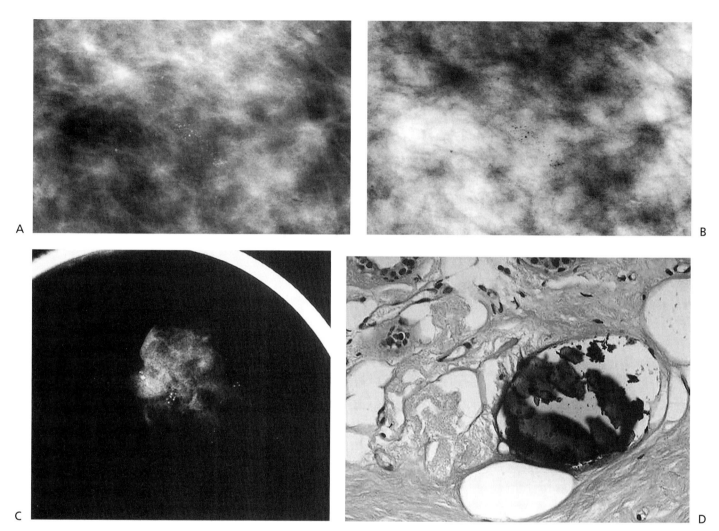

FIGURE 12-16. (A) Left breast, CC magnification view. **(B)** Inverted image of A. **(C)** Calcifications are present in the specimen radiograph. **(D)** The calcification is within a benign duct (H&E, 200×).

Findings

Predominately punctuate calcifications that appear to extend along a duct are seen. The image can be manipulated to display the calcifications as black dots on a light background. Their morphology and extent sometimes can be better evaluated with this technique.

A stereotactic core biopsy of this suspicious finding was performed.
Calcifications are present in the specimen radiograph (Fig. 12-16C).

Histology

Dystrophic calcifications in benign ducts (Fig. 12-16D).

Comment

The differential diagnosis for these types of calcifications includes low-grade ductal carcinoma in situ, fibrocystic change, and sclerosing adenosis with or without atypia.

When performing a stereotactic core biopsy of calcifications, a specimen radiograph of the sample should be obtained. This documents that calcifications have been sampled. If the pathology report does not mention calcifications, then the pathologist should be contacted to review the slides to look for them, or a radiograph of the paraffin block can be done to document that calcifications are present before additional sectioning of the tissue.

CASE 17

35-year-old female, 1-year status–post right lumpectomy and radiation therapy.

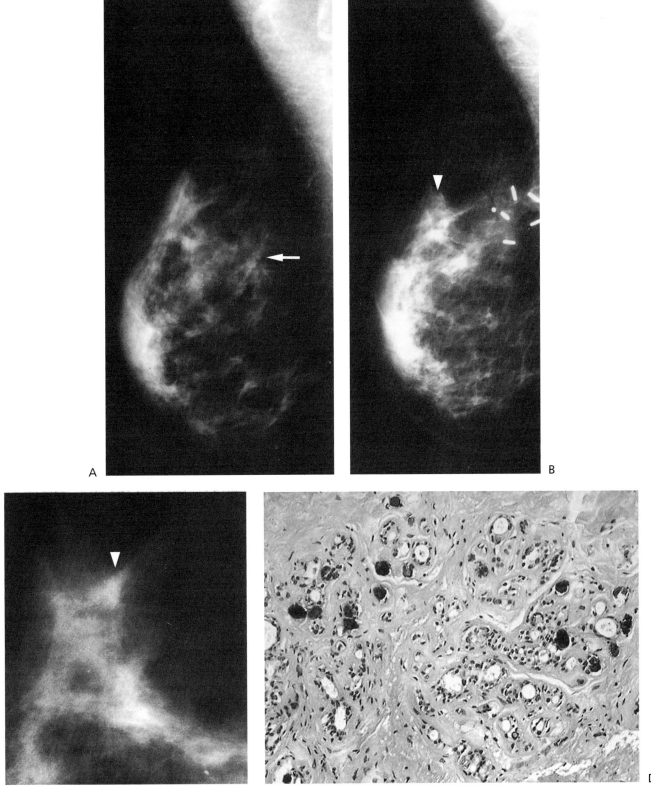

FIGURE 12-17. **(A)** Right breast, MLO view, screen-film study, 1 year earlier. **(B)** Right breast, MLO view, digital study, current. **(C)** 90-degree magnification view 4-cm anterior to the lumpectomy site, digital. **(D)** Numerous calcifications are present (H&E, 100×).

Findings

The initial mammogram demonstrates a 1.5-cm mass (*arrow* in Fig. 12-17A), which represented a 1.2-cm invasive ductal carcinoma.

The current study shows the posttreatment breast changes: overall increased density, surgical architectural distortion, and skin thickening.

A smaller than 1-cm cluster of amorphous calcifications (*arrowhead* in Fig. 12-17B and 12-17C) without associated features is seen anteriorly to the lumpectomy site. A stereotactic core biopsy was performed to exclude low-grade ductal carcinoma in situ.

Histology

Fibrocystic changes with associated calcifications, as seen in Figure 12-17D.

Comment

It is important to evaluate the whole breast and not just the lumpectomy site to exclude additional foci of malignancy in patients at risk for recurrence.

CASE 18

69-year-old female, history of cysts.

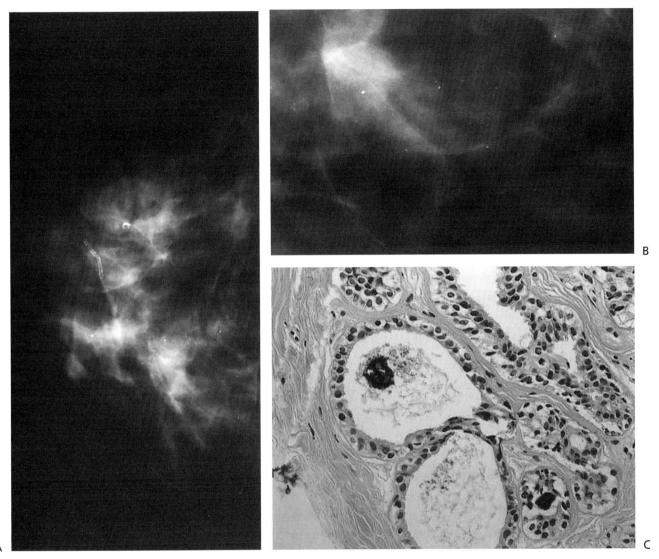

FIGURE 12-18. (A) Right breast, CC view. **(B)** CC magnification view. **(C)** Calcifications are present (H&E, 200×).

Findings

Calcifications are present in a segmental distribution in the medial aspect of the breast. The calcifications are variable in size, shape, and density. Several of the calcifications are linear in appearance. A stereotactic core biopsy was performed. It demonstrated fibrocystic changes and atypical ductal hyperplasia associated with calcifications. Because of the atypia on the core biopsy, a surgical excision was performed.

Histology

Proliferative fibrocystic changes and atypical ductal hyperplasia with associated calcifications are present in Figure 12-18C. No carcinoma was identified.

Comment

Segmental distribution of calcifications is a suspicious finding when the morphology of the calcifications is not specifically benign. This suggests the possibility of multifocal cancer.

CASE 19

72-year-old female, history of cysts.

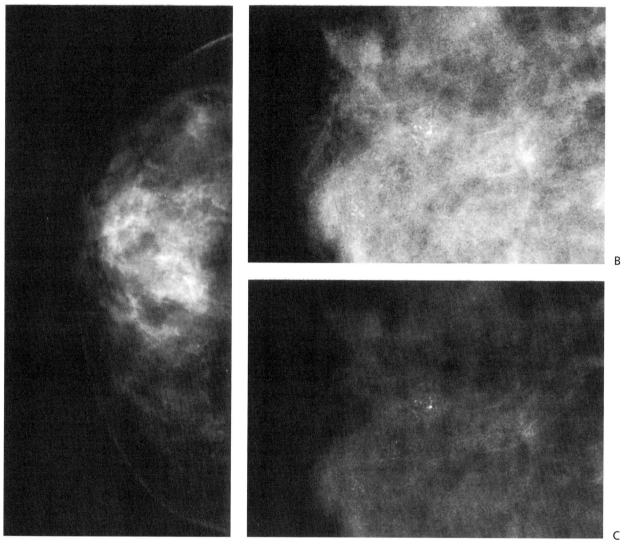

FIGURE 12-19. (A) Right breast, CC view. **(B,C)** CC magnification view of the subareolar region with different windowing and leveling of the image. **(D)** Inverted view of **B**. **(E)** The calcifications are associated with both processes (H&E, 40×).

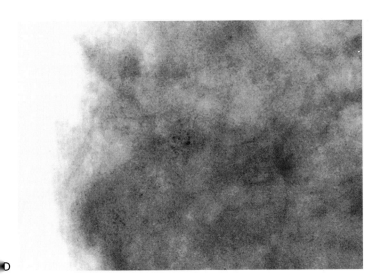

D

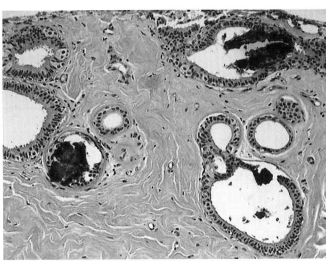

E

Findings

A faint cluster of calcifications is present in the subareolar region. The calcifications had increased in number and size when compared to previous studies (not shown). The magnification view demonstrates numerous amorphous and punctate calcifications without associated features. The extent of the calcifications is better appreciated on the inverted image.

Surgical excision of the suspicious calcifications was performed because these calcifications were too faint and located too far anteriorly, to be sampled with stereotactic guidance.

Histology

Mild intraductal hyperplasia with atypia and associated dystrophic calcifications in benign ducts (Fig. 12-19E).

Comment

Softcopy display systems can offer increased conspicuity of calcifications through manipulation of the images. The extent of the calcifications is also best appreciated on the contrast inverted image in this case.

CASE 20

46-year-old female, asymptomatic.

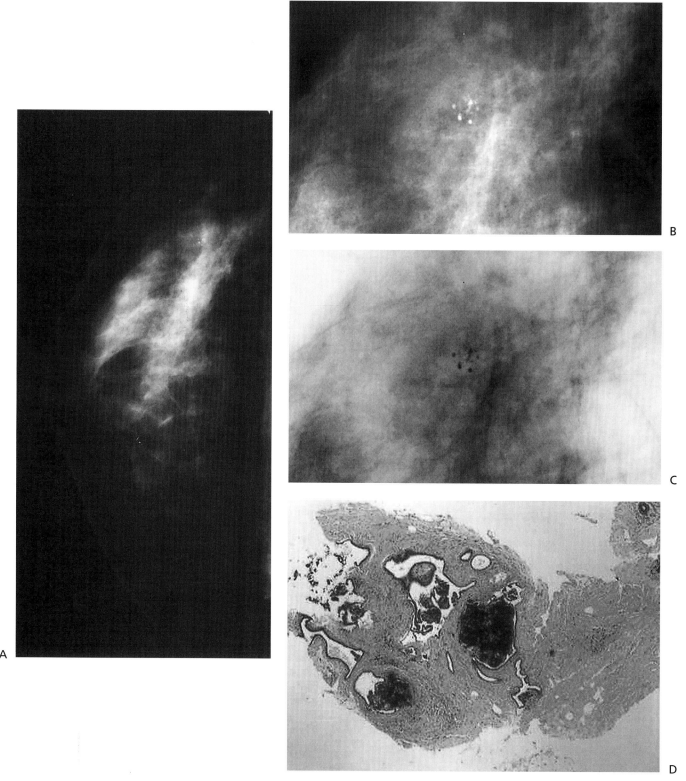

FIGURE 12-20. (A) Right breast, CC view. **(B)** CC magnification view. **(C)** Inverted image of **B**. **(D)** The calcifications are easily seen in one of the core biopsy samples (H&E, 20×).

Findings

On the standard view, a 1-cm cluster of calcifications is present in the lateral aspect of the breast posteriorly. The calcifications vary in size, shape, and density (pleomorphic).

This suspicious cluster was sampled with stereotactic guidance. The cluster had to be targeted with the inverted image because it was difficult to see the cluster on the dense breast parenchyma.

Histology

Small intraductal papilloma and calcifications associated with benign epithelium (Fig. 12-20D).

Comment

Intermediate and high-grade ductal carcinoma in situ, fibrocystic change, fibroadenoma, and papilloma can present as pleomorphic calcifications. Biopsy is necessary for diagnosis.

CASE 21

55-year-old female, history of benign biopsies.

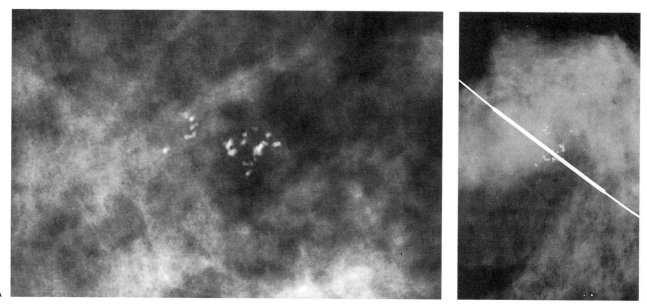

FIGURE 12-21. **(A)** Right breast, 90-degree magnification view. **(B)** Specimen radiograph of the calcifications.

Findings

Two clusters of coarse, dystrophic calcifications without a definite mass are present. Mammographically, these represent hyalinized fibroadenomas. Even with reassurance of the benign findings, the patient wanted these removed surgically, specimen radiograph (Fig. 12-21B).

Histology

Fibroadenomas.

Conclusion

Benign calcifications.

CASE 22

40-year-old female, 5-years status–post right lumpectomy and radiation therapy.

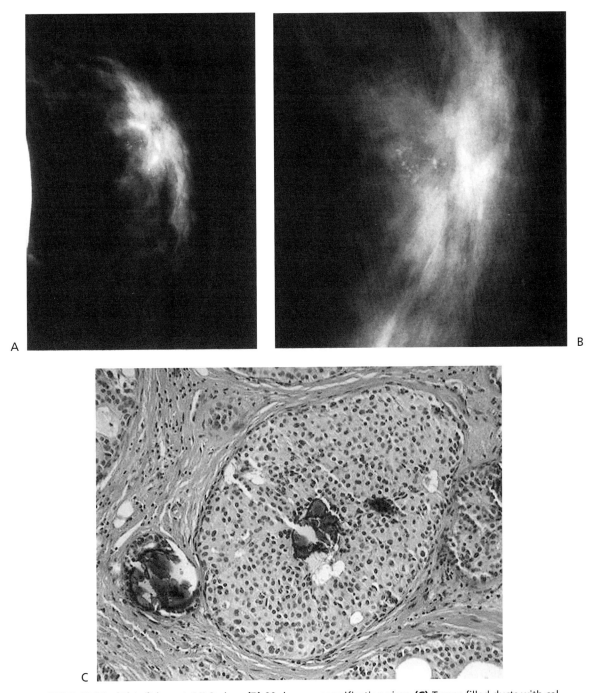

FIGURE 12-22. (A) Left breast, MLO view. **(B)** 90 degree magnification view. **(C)** Tumor filled ducts with calcifications (H&E, 100×).

Findings

A 1-cm cluster of calcifications is seen in the subareolar region of the breast, 4-cm from the nipple. Note the silicone implant posteriorly in this implant displaced-view.

The calcifications are pleomorphic (different sizes, shapes, and densities). Some of the calcifications are linear in appearance with ductal orientation. The architectural distortion anteriorly to the cluster is the patient's lumpectomy site. For diagnosis, a stereotactic core biopsy of the suspicious calcifications was performed.

Histology

Ductal carcinoma in situ, comedo-type with necrosis (Fig. 12-22C).

Comment

The patient underwent a simple mastectomy that showed 1.5-cm of ductal carcinoma in situ without invasion.

CASE 23

77-year-old female, asymptomatic.

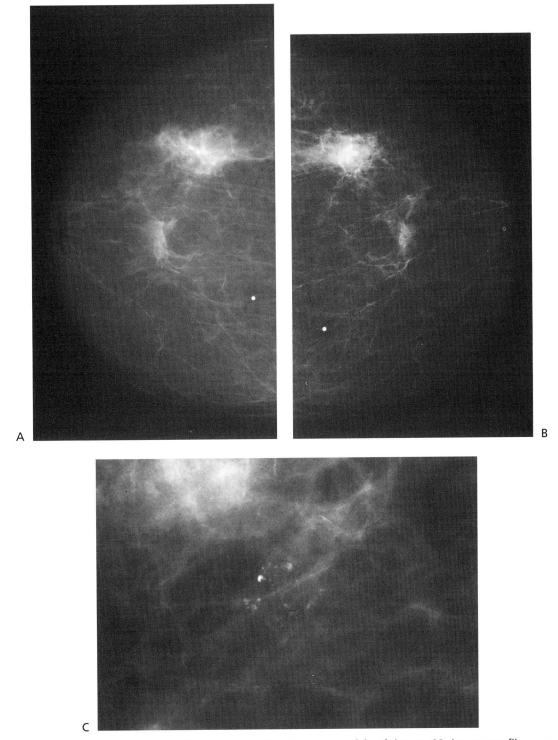

FIGURE 12-23. (A) Left breast, CC view, screen-film, 3 years prior. **(B)** Left breast, CC view, screen-film, current study. **(C)** CC magnification view, digital. **(D)** Calcifications are present in the specimen radiograph obtained after the stereotactic biopsy. **(E)** Localized pleomorphic calcifications.

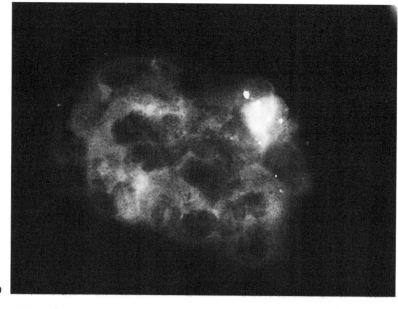

D

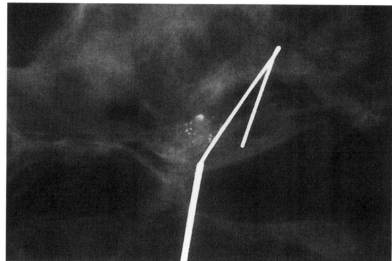

E

Findings

A new cluster of calcifications is present in the lateral aspect of the breast. This cluster is pleomorphic, without associated findings. Because the cluster is suspicious, a stereotactic core biopsy was performed. Calcifications are present in the specimen radiograph obtained after the stereotactic biopsy (Fig. 12-23B). Microscopically, fibrocystic changes and atypical ductal hyperplasia were present. Both were associated with the calcifications.

A surgical excision was performed. The localized pleomorphic calcifications are present in the specimen radiograph (Fig. 12-23C). Also, the density seen lateral to the calcifications in Figure 12-23C was removed, and it represented fibrocystic changes.

Histology

Ductal carcinoma in situ, solid subtype without necrosis, 0.5-cm, and sclerosing adenosis.
Both were associated with calcifications.

Comment

Any time that atypia is the diagnosis on a core biopsy, either for calcifications or a mass, surgical excision should be recommended because of the possibility of initial sampling error, such as occurred in this case.

CASE 24

64-year-old female, asymptomatic.

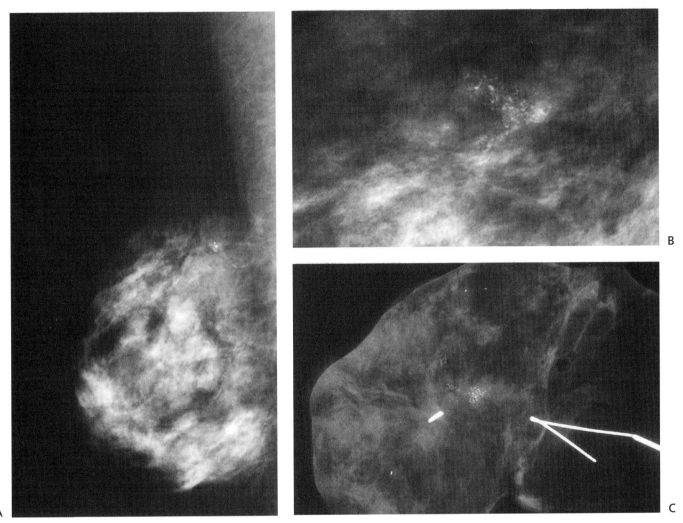

FIGURE 12-24. **(A)** Right breast, MLO view. **(B)** 90-degree magnification view. **(C)** The cluster of calcifications is present in the surgical specimen radiograph.

Findings

Two clusters of calcifications are present in the superior aspect of the breast.

The posterior cluster represents a hyalinized fibroadenoma. The anterior cluster (Fig. 12-24B) is mildly pleomorphic (granular) in appearance.

A stereotactic guided core biopsy of the suspicious cluster demonstrated 0.2-cm of ductal carcinoma in situ, cribriform pattern without necrosis, and associated with calcifications.

Breast conservation surgery was performed and the cluster of calcifications is present in the surgical specimen radiograph (Fig. 12-24C).

Histology

Sclerosing adenosis with associated calcifications at open biopsy.

No in situ or invasive cancer was seen. The entire malignancy was removed at core biopsy.

Comment

Granular calcifications have about a 20% risk of malignancy and should be sampled.

CASE 25

55-year-old female, asymptomatic.

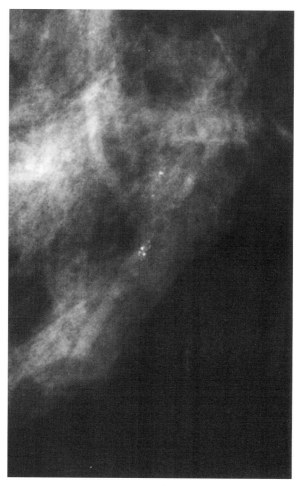

FIGURE 12-25. Left breast, 90-degree magnification view.

Findings

Several clusters of pleomorphic calcifications are seen. The largest two were sampled with stereotactic guidance.

Histology

Ductal carcinoma in situ, solid and cribriform without necrosis, was present at both locations, and both were associated with the calcifications.

Comment

At the time of the patient's lumpectomy, the clusters were bracketed with localization wires to help ensure complete removal of this area by the surgeon. The patient had multifocal ductal carcinoma in situ.

CASE 26

58-year-old female, asymptomatic.

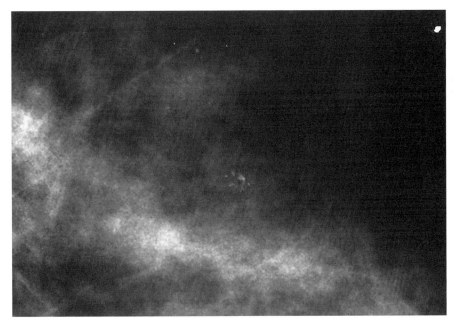

FIGURE 12-26. Left breast, 90-degree magnification view.

Findings

A 0.5-cm cluster of predominately round to oval calcifications is present with a possible low-density mass. A 6-month follow-up was recommended to the patient. The patient wanted the area sampled. A stereotactic core biopsy was done.

Histology

Ductal carcinoma in situ, micropapillary subtype without necrosis, and associated with calcifications.

Comment

Even relatively benign appearing calcifications can be malignant sometimes.

CASE 27

56-year-old female, asymptomatic.

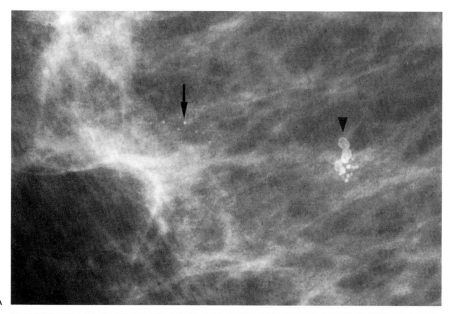

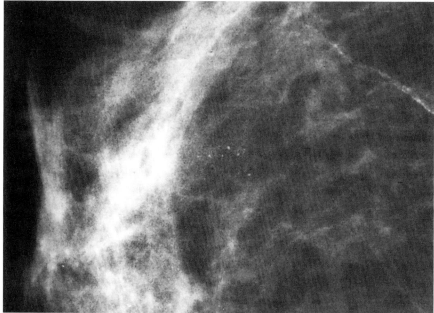

FIGURE 12-27. (A) Right breast, 90-degree magnification view. **(B)** Right breast, CC magnification view.

Findings

In Figure 12-27A, benign calcifications (*arrowhead*) are noted posteriorly. Predominately round, ductally oriented calcifications (*arrow*) are seen anteriorly in Figure 12-27A. Nevertheless, the anterior calcifications are mildly pleomorphic and remain ductally oriented, as seen in Figure 12-27B. A stereotactic core biopsy of the suspicious anterior calcifications was performed.

Histology

Ductal carcinoma in situ, micropapillary subtype without necrosis, but associated with the calcifications.

Comment

As with a mass, calcifications need to be evaluated in more than one projection and classified by its most worrisome features.

CASE 28

Two different patients.

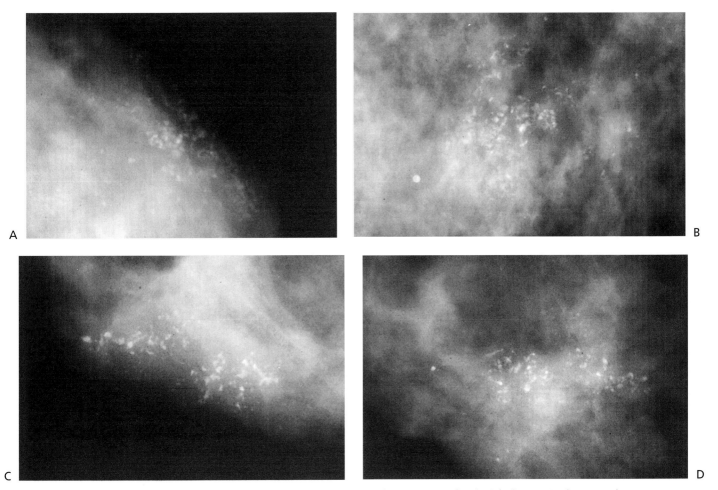

FIGURE 12-28. (A,B) Left breast, 90-degree and CC magnification views. **(C,D)** Right breast, 90-degree and CC magnification views.

Findings

Extensive pleomorphic calcifications are present. Some of the calcifications are linear and branching in appearance.

Histology

Ductal carcinoma in situ, comedo subtype with necrosis.

Comment

Even though the calcifications appear coarse, their pleomorphism is worrisome, and they should never be confused with benign calcifications.

CASE 29

39-year-old female, history of cysts.

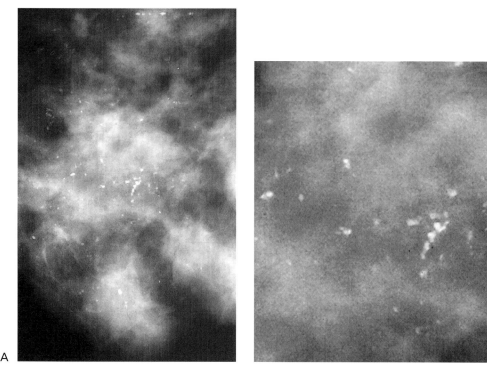

FIGURE 12-29. (A) Right breast, 90-degree view enlarged. **(B)** 90-degree magnification view.

Findings

Ductally oriented calcifications which are highly suggestive of malignancy are present in the central portion of the image. Also identified are extensive scattered pleomorphic calcifications. The oval/round masses proved to be cysts at ultrasound.

Histology

Ductal carcinoma in situ, comedo and solid subtypes with necrosis.

Comment

Whenever a patient has diffuse calcifications, it is important to assess all of them carefully for clusters that are not typical for the overall pattern seen elsewhere. In this case, the ductally oriented calcifications are easily appreciated. The other suspicious calcifications may have been less obvious at first glance. However, evaluation of the rest of both breasts is important to evaluate for other abnormalities. The patient had multicentric disease without invasion.

CASE 30

79-year-old female, asymptomatic.

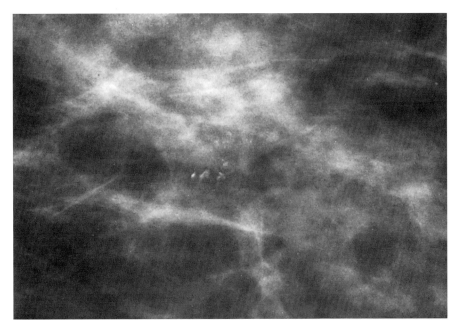

FIGURE 12-30. Left breast, 90-degree magnification view.

Findings

A cluster of pleomorphic calcifications is present. Note the "V-shaped" and linear types.

Histology

Ductal carcinoma in situ, solid and comedo subtypes with necrosis.

CASE 31

58-year-old female, asymptomatic.

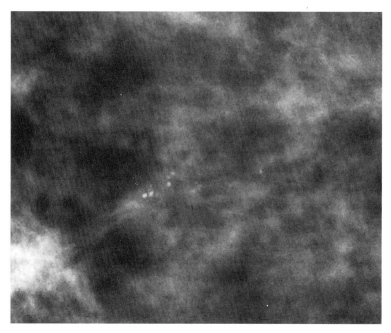

FIGURE 12-31. Left breast, CC magnification view.

Findings

A less than 1-cm cluster of pleomorphic (granular-type) calcifications is present.

Histology

Ductal carcinoma in situ, comedo subtype.

Comment

Note the 1-cm, spiculated, high-density mass posterior to the calcifications. This was an invasive ductal carcinoma. It is important to look for other abnormalities because the presence of more than one lesion may change the patient's treatment.

CASE 32

42-year-old female, status–post right mastectomy.

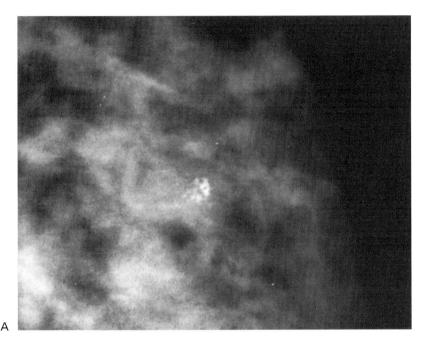

A

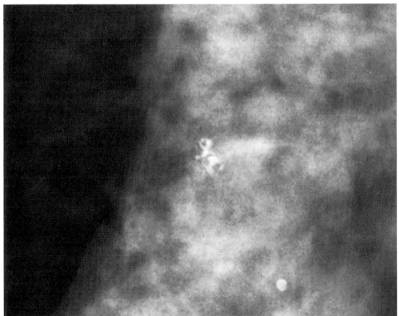

B

FIGURE 12-32. (A) Left breast, 90-degree magnification view. **(B)** Left breast, CC magnification view.

Findings

A cluster of calcifications that appears predominately coarse in nature is seen. A stereotactic core biopsy was performed.

Histology

Ductal carcinoma in situ, comedo subtype with necrosis.

CASE 33

Different patients.

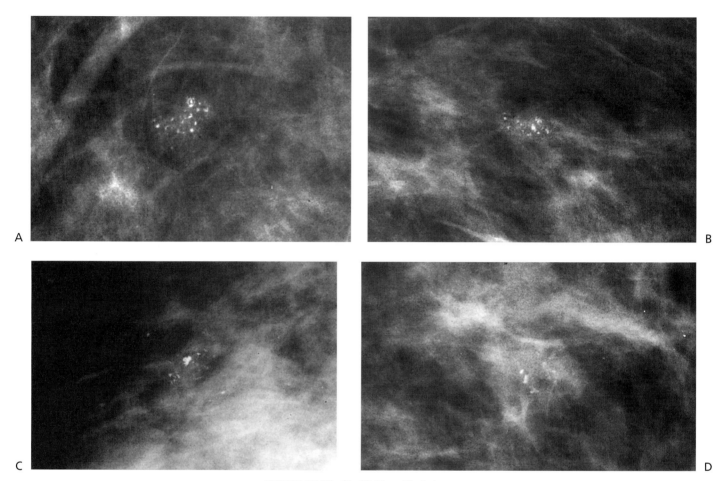

FIGURE 12-33. (A–D) Magnified views.

Findings

A pleomorphic cluster of calcifications is seen in each case without associated findings. Note that some of the calcifications are angulated and V-shaped. All of these clusters are suspicious for malignancy.

Histology

Case A & C: Ductal carcinoma in situ, comedo and solid subtypes with necrosis, associated with calcifications.
Case C & D: Fibroadenoma with associated calcifications.

Comment

These cases all demonstrate suspicious calcifications for which biopsy is needed.

CASE 34

60-year-old female, asymptomatic.

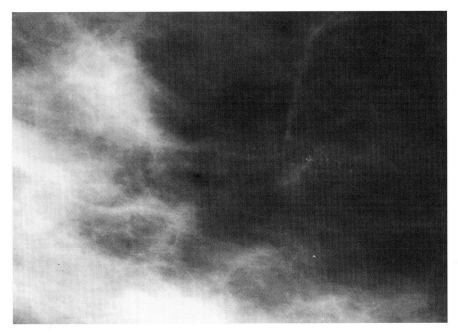

FIGURE 12-34. Right breast, CC magnification view.

Findings

Round, punctate, and fine linear calcifications are present in a ductal orientation with a possible associated density. A stereotactic core biopsy was performed for diagnosis.

Histology

Ductal carcinoma in situ, micropapillary subtype without necrosis, associated with calcifications.

Comment

Besides the morphology of the calcifications, their distribution is also important.

CASE 35

45-year-old female with a pulling sensation in lateral left breast.

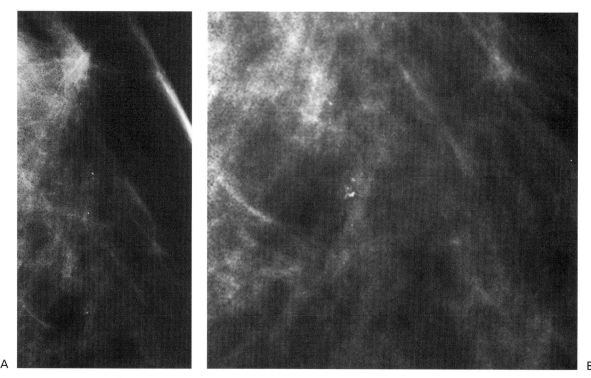

Figure 12-35. (A) Left breast, CC view enlarged. **(B)** CC magnification view.

Findings

A 1-cm, spiculated, high-density mass is easily seen. However, three tiny clusters of calcifications are present medial to it. They are pleomorphic in appearance. Core biopsies of the mass and the most medial cluster of calcifications were performed for diagnosis.

Histology

The mass proved to be invasive ductal carcinoma, well differentiated.
The calcification cluster was ductal carcinoma in situ, cribriform, and solid subtypes, without necrosis.

Comment

The mass, highly suggestive of malignancy, is obvious. However, one must look more carefully for the other abnormalities. Magnification views are important to characterize findings and to look for extent of disease. Because of the extent of disease in her breast, this patient opted for mastectomy.

CASE 36

68-year-old female, research screening study.

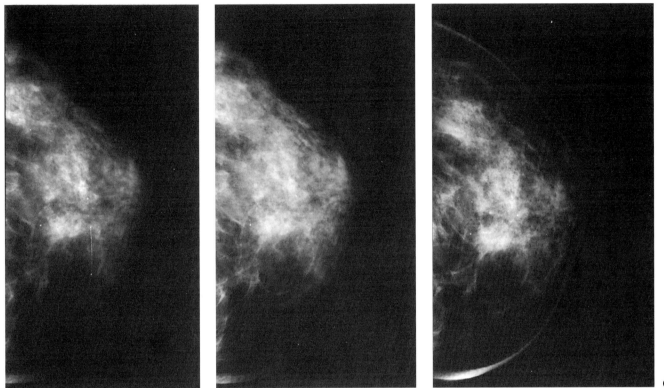

A,B   C

FIGURE 12-36. (A) Left breast, CC view, screen-film. **(B)** Left breast, CC view, digital (50-µm pixels, 10 bits/pixel). **(C)** Left breast, CC view, digital (100-µm pixels, 14 bits/pixel). **(D)** Left breast, CC magnification view, digital–same system as **C**. **(E)** Extensive calcifications. **(F)** Large ductal epithelial cells with high-grade nuclei, associated necrosis, and calcifications (H&E, 100×).

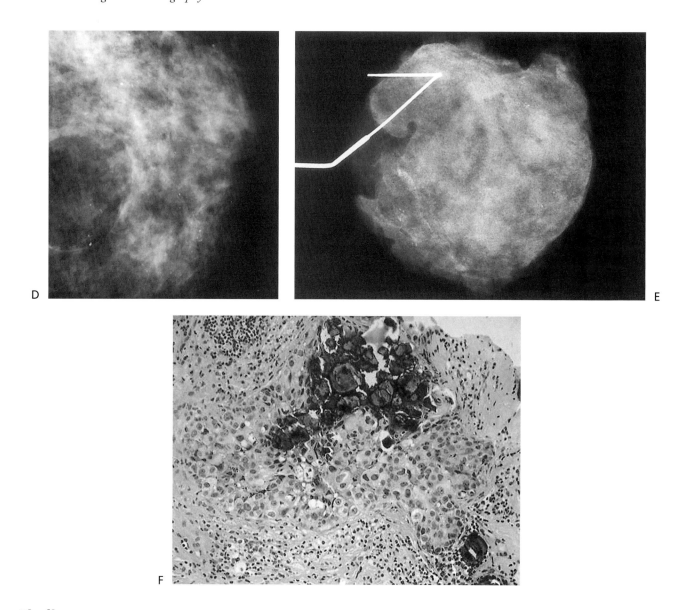

Findings

A 5 to 6-cm area of calcifications is present in the anterior and central subareolar region of the breast as seen in Figure 12-36A through 12-36D. The calcifications are clustered and scattered. Some of the calcifications are pleomorphic in appearance.

A stereotactic core biopsy was performed, and demonstrated ductal carcinoma in situ, solid and comedo subtypes with and without necrosis. The calcifications were associated with the in situ disease and benign epithelium. The patient underwent a surgical excision, and extensive calcifications are seen in the specimen radiograph (Fig. 12-36E).

Histology

Ductal carcinoma in situ, solid, cribriform, and comedo subtypes with necrosis, 5-cm with multiple positive margins (Fig. 12-36F).

Comment

The patient underwent a simple left mastectomy, which showed residual multicentric in situ disease. No invasive component was seen, and two sentinel lymph nodes were negative for metastatic involvement.

CASE 37

41-year-old female, history of mother with premenopausal breast cancer.

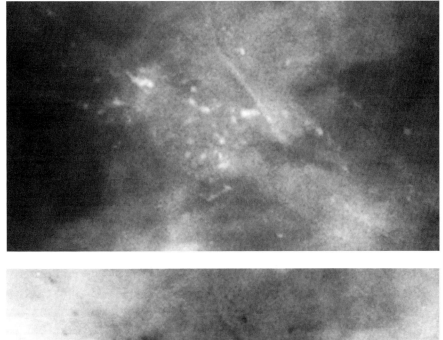

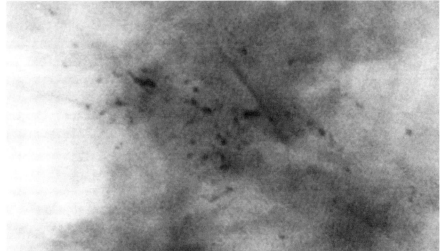

FIGURE 12-37. (A) Left breast, CC magnification view. **(B)** Contrast inversion view of **A**.

Findings

Ductally oriented casting and granular calcifications are present. No definite associated mass is seen. The extent of the calcifications is better visualized in the inverted image for some readers. A core biopsy was performed for diagnosis.

Histology

Ductal carcinoma in situ, comedo subtype with necrosis.

Comment

This case demonstrates malignant calcifications.

CASE 38

50-year-old female, 20-years status–post left lumpectomy for ductal carcinoma in situ.

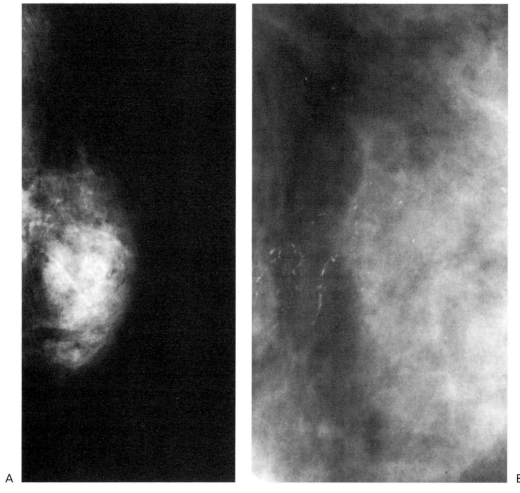

A

B

FIGURE 12-38. (A) Left breast, MLO view. **(B)** Left breast, 90-degree magnification view. **(C)** Surgical specimen radiograph. **(D)** Extensive necrosis is present (H&E, 20×).

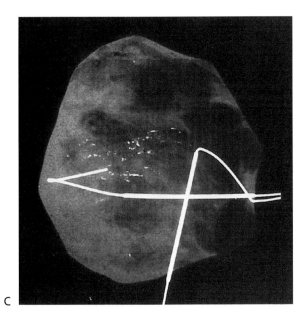

C

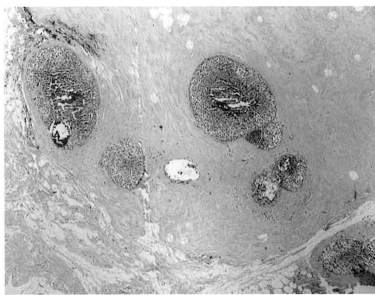

D

Findings

A 2 to 3-cm cluster of calcifications is seen in the posterior central part of the breast.

The calcifications are linear and branching in appearance. No associated mass is seen. A surgical excision was done. The morphology of the calcifications is well demonstrated in the specimen radiograph (Fig. 12-38C).

Histology

Ductal carcinoma in situ, comedo subtype with necrosis, 2.5-cm (Fig. 12-38D).

The patient underwent a salvage mastectomy, and 0.6-cm of residual DCIS was noted.

Comment

This case demonstrates mammographic findings highly suggestive of ductal carcinoma in situ, comedo subtype with necrosis.

CASE 39

58-year-old, asymptomatic female.

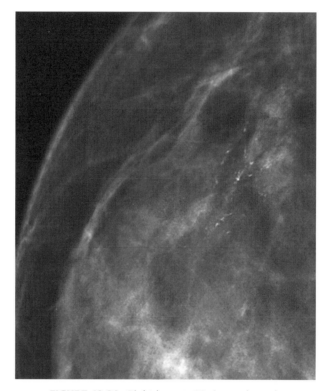

FIGURE 12-39. Right breast, CC view enlarged.

Findings

Extensive linear and branching (casting type) calcifications without associated features are present.

Conclusion

Mammographic findings highly suggestive of malignancy.

Histology

Ductal carcinoma in situ, comedo subtype with necrosis.

Comment

These calcifications represent comedo-type ductal carcinoma in situ with necrosis until proven otherwise.

CASE 40

62-year-old female, asymptomatic.

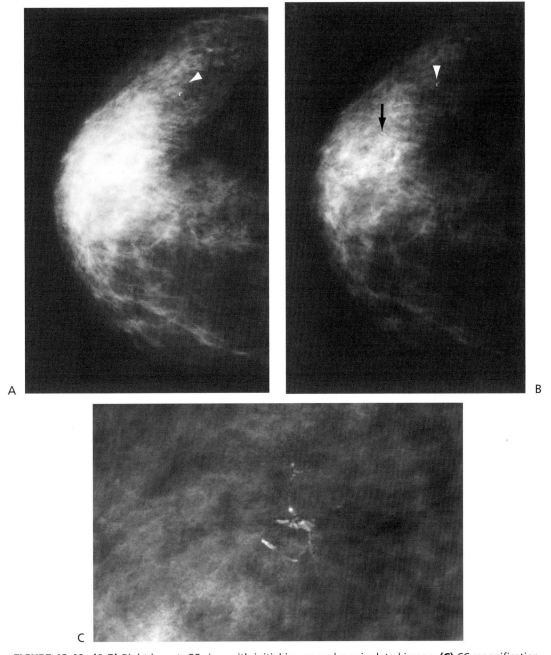

FIGURE 12-40. (A,B) Right breast, CC view with initial image and manipulated image. **(C)** CC magnification view of the anterior cluster. **(D)** Ductally oriented calcifications in the specimen radiograph. **(E)** Calcifications are associated with benign changes (H&E, 100×).

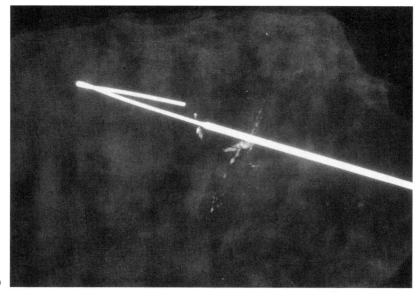

D

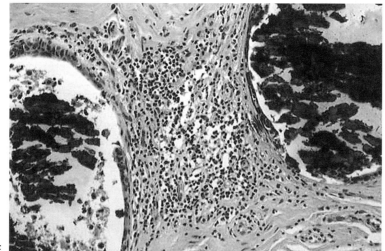

E

Findings

Two 1-cm clusters of calcifications are present in the lateral aspect of the breast. The posterior cluster (*arrowhead*) is dystrophic and easily visualized.

It is only with manipulation of the image on the softcopy display system that the anterior cluster (*arrow*) can be seen. Casting and pleomorphic calcifications are noted.

Since the patient could not tolerate a stereotactic core biopsy, a surgical excision was performed, and the ductally oriented calcifications are identified in the specimen radiograph (Fig. 12-40D).

Histology

Proliferative fibrocystic changes with associated dystrophic calcifications (Fig. 12-40E).

No malignancy was identified.

Comment

Given their morphology, it was surprising that these calcifications were benign. Classifying calcifications as benign or malignant is often challenging.

13

MISCELLANEOUS DIGITAL MAMMOGRAPHY

CHERIE M. KUZMIAK

CASE 1

42-year-old female with intermittent right breast pain.

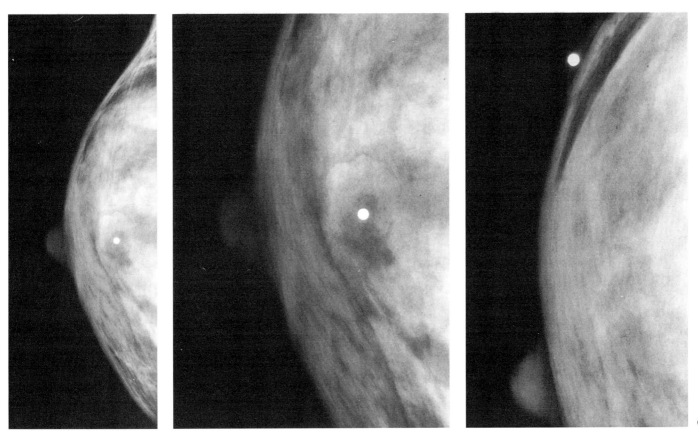

B

C

FIGURE 13-1. Right breast, CC view. **(A)** A metallic BB is placed on the patient's skin lesion. **(B)** CC view enlarged. **(C)** MLO view enlarged.

Findings

The skin lesion has a lobulated contour and is sharply outlined by air. The MLO view shows the raised skin lesion superiorly to the nipple.

Conclusion

Skin lesion.

Comment

Occasionally, a skin lesion can be confused mammographically with a mass in the breast. It is recommended that the technologist place a metallic marker on it prior to imaging to help avoid this problem.

CASE 2

45-year-old female, asymptomatic.

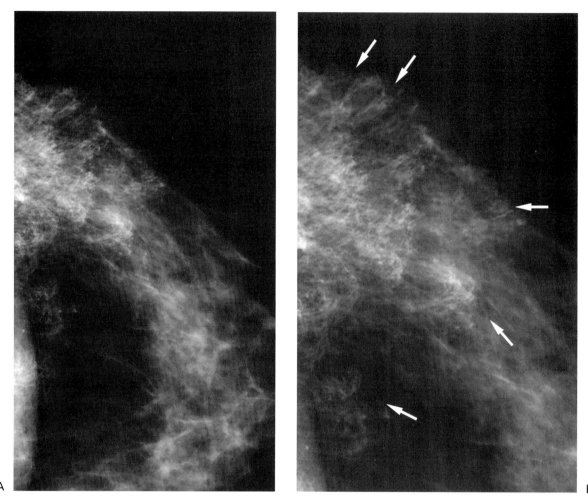

FIGURE 13-2. Right breast. **(A)** CC view laterally. **(B)** CC view enlarged.

Findings

Swirly, curvilinear densities (*arrows*).

Conclusion

This is an artifact from the patient's hair being projected over the breast during exposure of the image.

CASE 3

40-year-old female, asymptomatic.

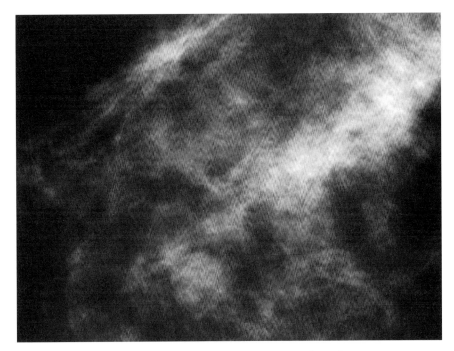

FIGURE 13-3. Right breast, CC view enlarged.

Findings

Thin black lines in a "zigzag" pattern.

Conclusion

This is an electronic interference artifact.

CASE 4

79-year-old male with a painful, palpable right breast mass.

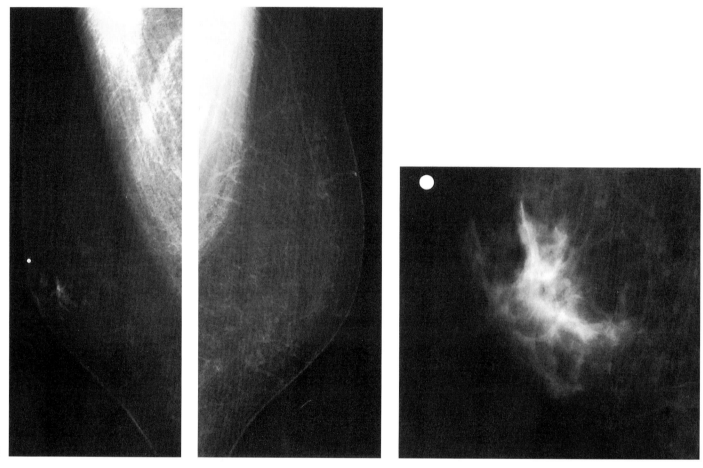

A,B

FIGURE 13-4. MLO views of **(A)** right breast and **(B)** left breast. A metallic BB marks the area of concern. **(C)** Right breast, MLO magnification view.

Findings

Normal glandular tissue is present in the subareolar region of the right breast. No mass or calcifications are seen on the magnification view. Normal fatty left breast.

Conclusion

Right breast gynecomastia.

Comment

Gynecomastia is a benign but painful condition. Peak incidences are at adolescence and older age. Causes include drugs (prescription and illicit), liver dysfunction, estrogen-producing testicular tumors, and idiopathic. This patient had no known cause.

CASE 5

37-year-old male with a painful right breast.

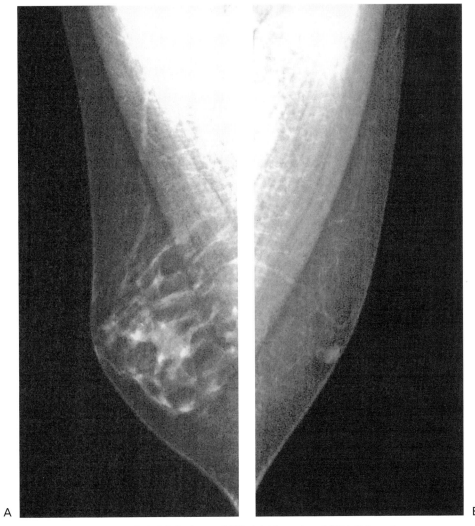

FIGURE 13-5. MLO views of **(A)** right breast and **(B)** left breast.

Findings

Diffuse glandular tissue is present in the right breast. No signs of malignancy are seen.
The left breast is normal.

Conclusion

Right breast gynecomastia.

Comment

The patient's gynecomastia was most likely secondary to his protease-inhibitor medications.

CASE 6

40-year-old female, asymptomatic.

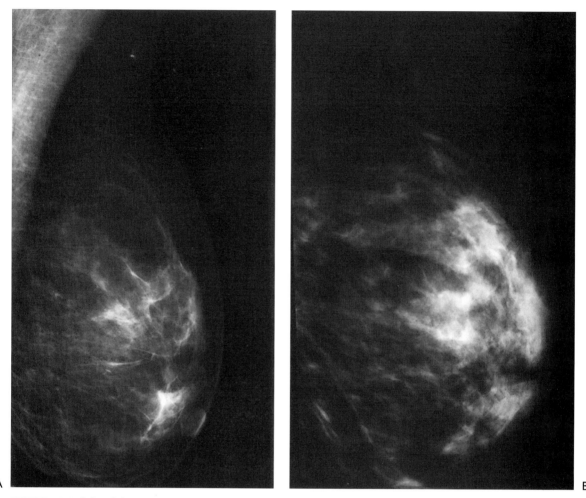

FIGURE 13-6. (A) Left breast, MLO view. **(B)** Left breast, MLO view, 2 years later when the patient is lactating.

Findings

The breast is heterogeneously dense and diffusely increased in density when compared to the nonlactating study.

Conclusion

Lactational changes.

Comment

If a mammogram has to be performed on a lactating patient, it is recommended that the patient breast-feed or use a breast pump immediately prior to imaging. This will help decrease the overall density of the breasts.

CASE 7

40-year-old female, history of implants.

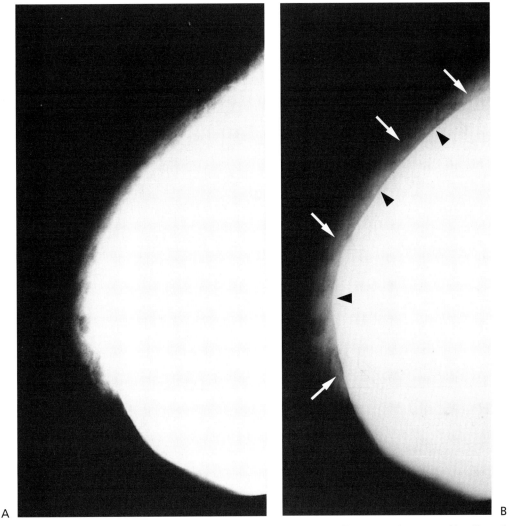

FIGURE 13-7. (A) Right breast, CC implant in-view, initial image. **(B)** Different windowing and leveling of **A**.

Findings

High-density material (*arrows* in Figure 13-7B) is seen external to the capsule of the implant (*arrowheads*) and is best seen in the second image. The high-density material is silicone.

Conclusion

Extracapsular rupture of a silicone implant.

Comment

The softcopy display system allows the reviewer to manipulate the image to evaluate the implant and, frequently, to see the extended silicone better.

CASE 8

56-year-old female, history of implants.

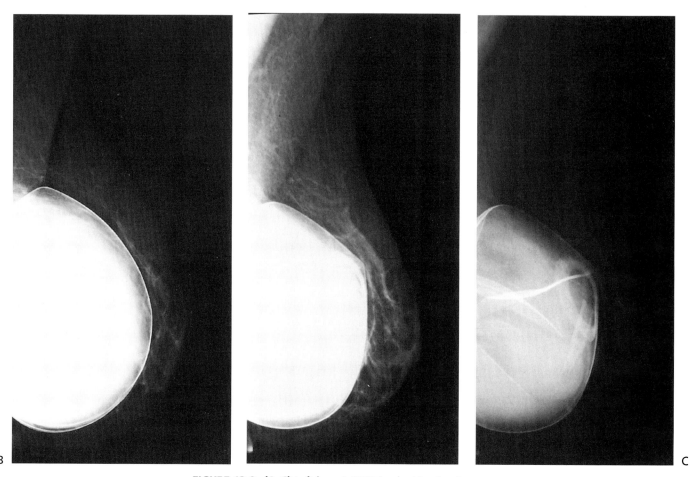

A,B   C

FIGURE 13-8. (A–C) Left breast, MLO implant in-view image.

Findings

A subglandular saline implant is shown. Figure 13-8A is the initial image. The image was manipulated with the softcopy display system to show the tissue anteriorly (Fig. 13-8B) and the implant (Fig. 13-8C), with its normal folds and valve.

Conclusion

Normal saline implant.

Comment

Saline implants are less dense mammographically than silicone implants, as can be seen in Case 7.

Even though the softcopy display system allows the reviewer to visualize the tissue anteriorly to the implant, implant displaced (pushed back) views are still indicated to evaluate the breast tissue optimally.

CASE 9

A 36-year-old female with right breast invasive ductal carcinoma was enrolled in a neoadjuvant study to downstage the tumor prior to lumpectomy. The patient had a significant clinical response after the first dose of chemotherapy (adriamycin and cytoxin). Before any further chemotherapy, the tumor was marked with a metallic marker.

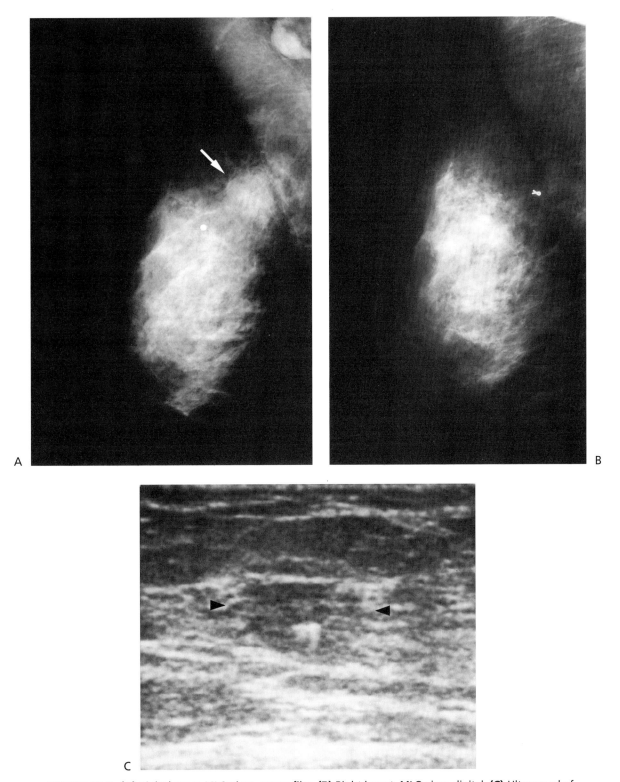

A

B

C

FIGURE 13-9. (A) Right breast, MLO view, screen-film. **(B)** Right breast, MLO view, digital. **(C)** Ultrasound of the mass (*arrowheads*) with the echogenic marker clip.

Findings

Figure 13-9A is the patient's original study with the malignant mass (*arrow* in Fig. 13-9A) located superiorly at the level of the pectoralis muscle. Note the suspicious lymph node in the axilla. Figure 13-9B is the postprocedure mammogram with the metallic clip in the mass. The mass is difficult to visualize mammographically. The isoechoic, irregular mass (*arrowheads*) with the echogenic marker clip is best seen on the ultrasound study (Fig. 13-9C).

Comment

In the setting of neoadjuvant therapy with planned breast conservation surgery, it is extremely important to place a metallic marker in or adjacent to the mass. If there is complete response to the chemotherapy, and the mass has not been marked, it is difficult to localize the area for surgery, whether the breast is dense or fatty in appearance.

After placement of a metallic marker, postprocedure mammograms are recommended for documentation of placement.

CASE 10

A 34-year-old female presents with a 3-day history of a tender, palpable mass medial to the nipple areolar complex. The patient had bilateral reduction mammoplasty 4 years ago.

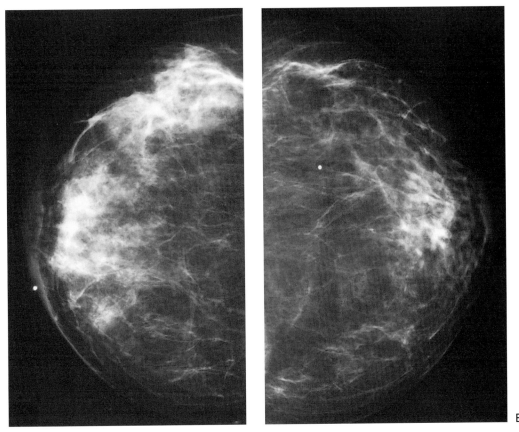

A   B

FIGURE 13-10. CC views of **(A)** right breast and **(B)** left breast. A metallic BB marks the area of patient concern. **(C)** Right breast, CC magnification view. **(D)** Left breast, CC view of the subareolar region enlarged. **(E)** Ultrasound of the patient's mass.

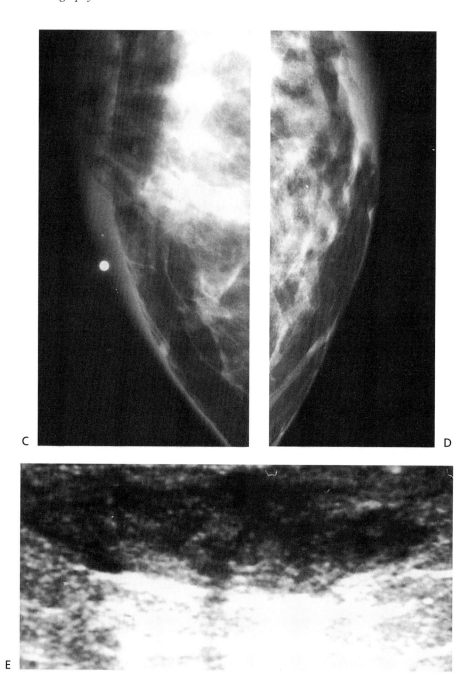

Findings

Focal skin thickening is noted beneath the BB in the right breast. Notice how thickened it is when compared to the normal skin line of the left breast. No discrete mass is seen in either breast. Only asymmetric breast tissue is present.

Sonographically, the patient's mass represents a 3-cm, heterogeneous, horizontally oriented lesion in the skin. Under real-time ultrasound, mobile debris was seen in the mass (Fig. 13-10E).

Histology

Abscess, with acute and chronic inflammation.

Comment

With post-processing algorithms and the ability to manipulate the images with the digital softcopy display system, the skin and subcutaneous regions are easier to evaluate. The skin can be seen on screen-film mammography, but the film usually has to be placed over a "hot-light" to view it.

CASE 11

82-year-old female treated with a right lumpectomy and radiation therapy 1 year ago.

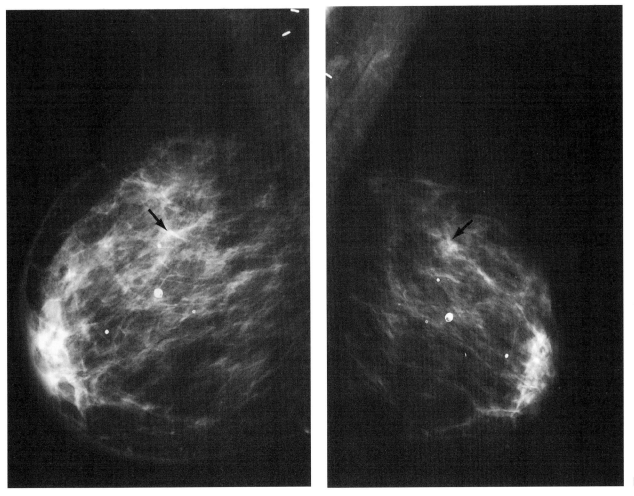

A   B

FIGURE 13-11. Both of the images were obtained on the same day. **(A)** Right breast, MLO view, digital. **(B)** Right breast, MLO view, screen-film.

Findings

Skin and parenchymal thickening is present. These findings are better visualized in the digital study. Subtle architectural distortion is visualized superiorly at the patient's lumpectomy site (*arrow*).

Conclusion

Posttreatment findings.

Comments

Mastitis, inflammatory breast cancer, edema from lymphatic obstruction, and trauma are also in the differential diagnosis for this appearance. Knowledge of the patient's clinical history is important.

CASE 12

69-year-old female with swelling and erythema of the right breast.

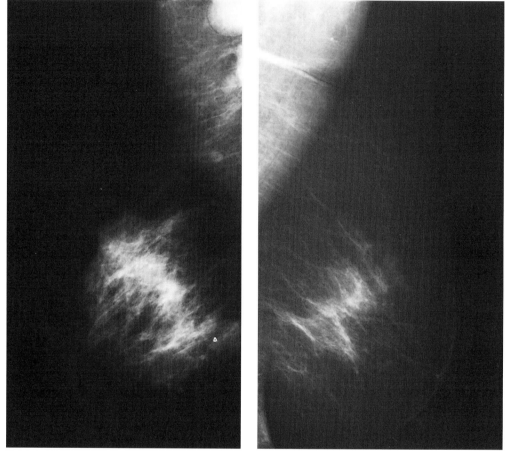

A

B

FIGURE 13-12. MLO views of **(A)** right breast and **(B)** left breast. Enlarged MLO views of the subareolar regions of **(C)** right breast and **(D)** left breast.

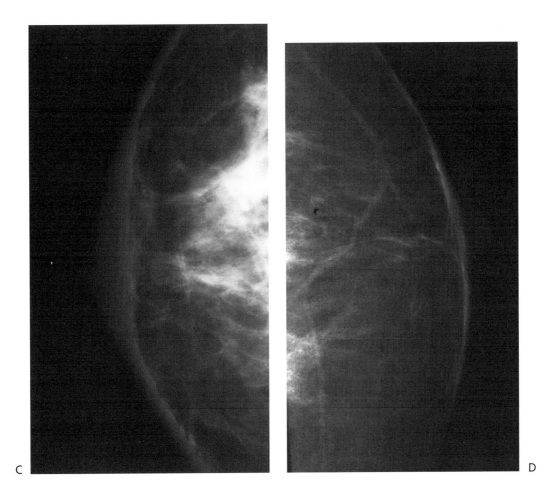

C   D

Findings

The entire right breast is abnormal. It is diffusely increased in density with parenchymal thickening. It is smaller in size and less compressible than the left. An irregular mass is visualized in the inferior aspect of the right breast at the site of a metallic marker clip. Abnormal skin thickening is present and is better appreciated when compared to the normal skin line of the left breast. Also note the abnormally dense right axillary lymph nodes. The left breast is normal.

Histology

Invasive ductal carcinoma, poorly differentiated, with dermal involvement and metastatic involvement of the lymph nodes.

Conclusion

Inflammatory breast carcinoma of the right breast.

Comments

If the breast is dense, the skin line may not be clearly seen on the initial image, even on a digital mammogram. Softcopy image manipulation may be needed to appreciate this finding.

SUBJECT INDEX

SUBJECT INDEX